THE

BRAN PLAN DIET

THE
BRAN
PLAN
DIET

OLIVER ALABASTER, M.D. & JANIS JIBRIN, R.D.

Rodale Press, Emmaus, Pennsylvania

Cover Design by Acey Lee

If you have any questions or comments concerning this book, please write:
Rodale Press
Book Readers' Service
33 East Minor Street
Emmaus, PA 18098

Library of Congress Cataloging-in-Publication Data

Alabaster, Oliver.
 The bran plan diet / by Oliver Alabaster & Janis Jibrin.
  p.   cm.
 Includes index.
 ISBN 0-87596-162-2 hardcover
 1. Reducing diets. 2. Bran. I. Jibrin, Janis II. Title.
RM222.2.A372 1993
613.2'5—dc20   92-29971
                                                              CIP

Distributed in the book trade by St. Martin's Press

2 4 6 8 10 9 7 5 3 1 hardcover

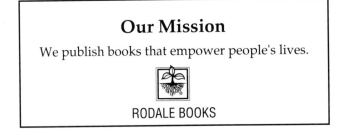

Our Mission
We publish books that empower people's lives.

RODALE BOOKS

Notice

This book is intended as a reference volume only, not as a medical guide or manual for self-treatment. If you suspect you have a medical problem, please seek competent medical care. Keep in mind that nutritional needs vary from person to person, depending upon age, sex, health status and total diet. The foods discussed and recipes given here are designed to help you make informed decisions about your diet and health. They are not intended as a substitute for any treatment prescribed by your doctor. Finally, if you have reason to believe that you might be allergic to psyllium, do not include it in the Bran Cocktail.

To my remarkable friend Dr. Denis Burkitt, whose extraordinary insight, originality and enthusiasm have influenced so many doctors to recognize both the importance of dietary fiber in promoting good health and the critical importance of adopting a preventive approach to health care.
—Oliver Alabaster

To Barbara Jibrin, an energetic and intelligent researcher.
—Janis Jibrin

Contents

C　　H　　A　　P　　T　　E　　R

1

Introducing
the Bran Plan Diet

You bought this book because you, like so many Americans, want to take control of your diet and your health. By now most of you know that nutrition affects not only body weight and appearance but also your energy level and how long you live. *The Bran Plan Diet* shows you how to gain complete control over what you eat and the way you eat. You'll learn how to lose excess weight and keep it off for good, how to have more energy than ever before and how to take your best shot at enjoying a longer, disease-free life.

So if you want to set your diet straight once and for all, the Bran Plan is the most vital and effective eating system available today. This plan, which is based upon the latest nutrition information science has to offer, will do two very important things for you.

- Provide you with the ultimate weight-control program that enables you to take off as many pounds as you need to, and even more important, keep them off permanently.

- Lead you into a lifelong eating plan in which you use foods that not only help you achieve your weight goals but also reduce your risk of heart disease, cancer and many other diseases associated with the typical American diet.

The Bran Plan equips you with a unique and very important tool for gaining the figure and glowing good health you desire: the Bran Cocktail. Like fruit cocktail, the Bran Cocktail is not a drink. This virtually calorie-free formula is a blend of various brans created to provide a balance of the types of fiber scientific researchers deem vital for keeping our bodies at their best. By simply sprinkling a small amount of the Bran Cocktail on appropriate foods throughout the day, you upgrade your diet by adding fiber and you feel much more satisfied with fewer calories. At the same time, you methodically add more fruits and vegetables to your menu plan, displacing undesirable foods that can cause weight gain and illness when eaten in excess. (See page 30 for a full description of the Bran Cocktail.)

We are confident that we can help you look and feel better because in designing the Bran Plan, we have employed the latest scientific findings that reveal which foods work best for weight loss, weight control and a lifetime of health. The Bran Plan has also been designed to make the transition to a new healthy eating experience easy, enjoyable, interesting and *permanent*.

After living through the fad diets of the 1970s and 1980s, and after watching Oprah Winfrey lose impressive pounds on one of the risky liquid diets—and gain it all back—many people became disillusioned with dieting. Sure, these quick-fix diets can help you take off lots of weight fast, but you put it on again, even faster. Some folks become professional dieters, trying each new diet, losing and then gaining until their metabolisms are so out of whack that any new attempt at losing weight becomes very difficult and gaining weight very easy—in fact, inevitable! So yo-yoing—dieting and reducing followed by bingeing and gaining—has been the miserable lot of far too many Americans. No one ever sticks with any of the fad diets over the long run because these systems are so restrictive, never emphasizing the value of good eating habits that use familiar, likable foods as the road to achieving optimum weight.

The Bran Plan avoids this mistake. Instead of rushing you into this new way of eating for a week or two, then letting you slip back into old habits, the Bran Plan first shows you how to control your weight, then shows you how to change your habits gradually, easing you into a life-long healthy eating pattern. Here's how.

Phase One of the Bran Plan (described in chapter 4), *adds some fiber* to your regular diet in the form of the Bran Cocktail, plus one fruit and one vegetable. *You won't be giving anything up,* just adding the mix of different brans and some foods that will give you an instant fiber boost, along with additional vitamins and minerals that they contain.

Phase Two (introduced in chapter 6) is for those who need *a clearly defined weight-loss program.* In chapter 7 we give you menus that are designed to take off about three to five pounds every four weeks. The scientifically balanced menus must be followed carefully for four weeks at a time and the program continued until you reach your desired weight. But the menus are not rigid; we offer choices both in the foods you eat and when you eat them. We even offer a take-out foods plan for those of you who don't want to cook.

Phase Three (summarized in chapter 10) eases you into a *lifelong eating plan* that eliminates all the high-calorie excess fat from your diet and provides you with enough fiber for maximum health. About 35 percent of cancer cases and heart disease cases are traceable, in whole or in part, to the American diet of today! Abundant scientific evidence now proves that certain foods have the power to heal, to maintain a youthful heart and blood vessels and to keep your body metabolism healthy. Other foods have the power to do just the opposite—destroy your health, increase your weight and make life not only shorter, but miserable, too.

The third phase is not a weight-loss diet, it's a guide to gradually replacing unhealthy eating habits with healthy ones. No matter how long you've been making the kinds of wrong food choices that result in ballooning measurements, you'll maintain healthy, steady weight on this phase. But if you start to gain again, you can always go back to Phase Two.

Whether you're losing weight on Phase Two or maintaining your ideal weight on Phase Three, you'll find the Bran Plan the most enjoy-able, valuable diet ever—one that fits right in with your lifestyle and food tastes. Here's why.

You'll eat normal foods. There are no wheatgrass juice and food-combining taboos in this book. You'll eat the type of foods you like, such as pasta, tuna fish, salads, even red meat occasionally. You'll simply learn to adjust the amounts while enjoying the healthiest pasta dishes or preparing sandwiches with tuna fish salad low in fat or even walking away with the best salad bar choices. The Bran Plan is ideal for vegetarians, but if you're a fan of red meat, we'll show you how to work a small amount into a healthy diet.

You'll follow an uncomplicated food plan. Silly rules like "Don't eat after 6:30 P.M." or "You must have a grapefruit before each meal" not only have no scientific validity but are completely unrealistic as well. Many of us don't even get home by 6:30!

If you are retired and able to organize regular mealtimes, you can tailor the Bran Plan to suit your preferences. If you're a businesswoman who has to take an endless stream of clients to lunch, you'll learn what to order at the business lunch and what to eat when you finally get home so that it all fits into the Bran Plan. If you tend to run late in the morning and miss breakfast, we'll show you how to slip in this healthy meal when you're at your desk. No matter what your lifestyle, this book will accommodate you, minus any of the complicated and bogus "scientific rules" that appear in so many other diet books.

You'll have more energy than ever before. Diets that have you eating fruit all day or make you go on stressful fasts can leave you so weak and listless that you barely make it through the day. Even on Phase Two, the weight-loss part of the Bran Plan, we make sure you get enough calories and the proper balance of vitamins and minerals to keep you in top physical form with plenty of energy. Whether you love the high intensity and sweat of an aerobics workout or just the relaxation and solitude of a long walk, this diet program ensures that you'll have more than enough energy to do it.

Another reason you'll feel more energetic on the Bran Plan is that it's rich in complex carbohydrates and moderate in sugar. Complex carbohydrates such as bread, pasta, rice and cereal supply you with a steady stream of energy instead of the uneven highs and lows that result from eating lots of sugary foods. Dessert lovers, stay with us! There's room for sweets in the Bran Plan—but we help you control any excessive cravings.

If you want to start the Bran Plan this minute, go straight to chapter 4. You are about to get into your best shape ever. We're excited about the Bran Plan, and we can't wait to lead you through it!

2

The Healing and Slimming Power of Fiber

*O*ne of the great benefits of the Bran Plan is that it will immediately increase your intake of dietary fiber, that indigestible yet valuable part of whole grain cereals, bran cereals, fruits, vegetables and legumes (nuts, black beans and such). The amount of fiber you'll take in will do wonders for your waistline as well as your health and longevity. Most Americans don't eat nearly enough fiber, and this fiber deficiency can be traced to the fact that our diet has changed so much from the diet of our ancestors—the diet that made us what we are today.

Our bodies have a delicate metabolic balance that is the product of thousands of years of evolution in which the human body adapted itself to a diet that was about 85 percent derived from plants and only about 15 percent derived from animals. However, the typical American diet of today is composed of only about 30 percent plant products, with the other 70 percent being mostly composed of meat and dairy foods, which are usually high in fat and provide no fiber at all. This dramatic shift in eating habits is blamed for a tragic increase in cancer and heart disease in this century, especially among those of middle age and beyond. Many such cases, which account for about 80 percent of premature deaths and illness among Americans, could be avoided in the future if we were to adopt a lifelong high-fiber, low-fat diet—and also avoid smoking.

On the other hand, low-fiber, high-fat diets help to keep about one-third of all Americans obese. But diets high in fiber fill you up on satisfying, low-calorie, nutritious foods, so there is little room for fatty foods that go straight to your belly or thighs.

By making sure that you get enough fiber, and keeping fat low, the Bran Plan is not only a wonderful way to slim but also can really help reduce your risk of falling prey to a number of major illnesses. Of course, diseases are caused by a variety of factors, and dietary fiber is only one important aspect of a healthy diet, not an absolute guarantee of a long life free of disease—although it will surely contribute greatly to that goal.

You can't beat unrefined cereals as a source of dietary fiber. As long ago as the fifth century B.C., Hippocrates recognized the laxative action of whole meal bread. Before the high-grinding system of milling was introduced in eighteenth-century France, everybody ate only whole grains. Then the rich began to adopt expensive, refined white flour products as a mark of social superiority. By the end of the nineteenth century, improved refining techniques made low-fiber white bread available to people in most countries of the industrialized world. Physicians of the day approved the health value of this refined white wheat flour. In fact, many of them soon began prescribing its use as a remedy for diverticulosis, a type of bowel disease. We now know that whole grain flour, not refined flour, is best for patients with this ailment.

It is largely because of such misguided changes in our dietary habits during this century that we have seen a rapid increase in colon cancer, breast cancer, heart disease, diverticular bowel disease, varicose veins and gallstones. And the decrease in fiber intake, due to the steady decline in our consumption of whole grain breads and bran cereals, fruits, vegetables and legumes (nuts, beans and so forth), is probably the most important cause. Incredibly, our bread and cereal consumption has fallen to about 20 percent of what it was a hundred years ago; a trend that must be reversed.

Fortunately, not all physicians early in this century were blind to the health value of whole grains and fiber. Among the enlightened ones was Dr. John Harvey Kellogg, whose name lives on in the Kellogg Company of Battle Creek, Michigan. Later, the observations of Dr. Denis Burkitt provoked widespread scientific interest in fiber and its power to help prevent many common diseases that afflict people in the industrialized world. While living in tropical Africa, Dr. Burkitt noticed that nearly all the diseases that frequently occurred in England were extremely rare among the Africans. Although he saw many serious medical problems in this group that were associated with climate and poverty, diseases like breast and colon cancer, heart disease, stroke, diabetes, irritable bowel syndrome, hemorrhoids, varicose veins, gallstones and intestinal polyps, so widespread in America and Europe, were rare. This very important observation drew attention to the fact that diseases so familiar in economically advanced countries were seldom seen in more primitive societies, and the reasons for this were more likely to be related to diet and lifestyle than to anything else, including inherited tendencies.

On closer examination, Dr. Burkitt saw that the African diet was much lower in fat and much higher in fiber than the diet found in Europe and North America. In fact, the African diet was much closer to the diet that humans had evolved with for thousands of years. In other words, it was much more *natural*, and therefore, healthier. This conclusion was validated when the frequency of diseases among immigrants to America was compared to the frequency with which these diseases occurred in their countries of origin. Generally speaking, settlers acquire the disease patterns of the country they go to, and they usually leave behind the diseases associated with their homeland. All this points to environmental causes of disease as being much more important than any we inherit, and the most important environmental cause of all lies in the choice of the foods we eat.

Scientific evidence generally supports the idea that dietary fiber intake should help reduce our risk of disease. However, researchers point out that life in rich countries also means exposure to more stress, less physical activity, a higher calorie intake and more cigarette smoking, all of which can contribute to our disease risk.

Nevertheless, the results of a major study in Holland in 1982 tends to confirm the high fiber/good health connection. Among 871 middle-aged men who were followed for ten years, those on low-fiber diets were three times more likely to die from all causes than those men who consumed high-fiber diets. Obviously, the high-fiber Lifelong Bran Plan will put you on the right track!

All Fiber Is Not Alike

Fiber is found only in vegetable products, never in animal products. As noted earlier, it is the calorie-free, indigestible part of whole grain cereals, fruits and vegetables. There is no one thing that identifies dietary fiber. In fact, there are a number of different types of fiber, which can act on the body in different ways. From a practical point of view, it is easier to think of dietary fiber as a catchall phrase for two basic types of fiber: the *soluble* (pectins, gums and mucilages—plus slightly soluble lignin) and the *insoluble* (cellulose and hemicellulose).

Soluble and insoluble fibers usually are found together in most fiber-rich foods. However, the relative amount of each type varies, so that different cereals, fruits and vegetables contain varying mixtures of these fibers. Now there are food labels giving soluble and insoluble fiber, usually lumped together as "dietary fiber." Soluble fibers are the predominant type found, for example, in psyllium and oat bran cereal and in fruit such as apples. They work to lower blood cholesterol, if consumed regularly and in sufficient quantity. Some of these fibers can form gels when exposed to water, and this creates bulk. Others, like lignin, basically pass through the intestine unchanged because they cannot react with water.

In contrast, insoluble fibers, the dominant type found in wheat bran, also produce their effects by holding water, which also makes them swell. This increase in bulk speeds up the passage of intestinal contents, producing a laxative effect.

Fiber also increases bulk by stimulating the growth of certain bacteria that are naturally present in the bowel. Sometimes this causes flatulence, particularly among people who adopt high-fiber diets too rapidly. It's best to make these changes gradually, not only because it is more comfortable but also because it gives the body time to get used to the effects of a high-fiber diet.

How Extra Bran Can Help Prevent Heart Attacks and Strokes

The main cause of death in the United States and in all the industrialized countries (provided the very elderly are included in the statistics) is heart disease. If we look only at the causes of dying prematurely (before the age of 70), however, cancer and heart disease are about equal. In any case, each of these health problems is a much greater threat to the health of the average American than a disease such as AIDS, which attracts far more publicity.

High cholesterol and heart disease. As you might expect by now, heart disease is much less common in poorer countries where people have to "make do" with a diet much lower in fat and higher in fiber than ours. Risk factors for heart disease include smoking, lack of exercise, being severely overweight and consuming too many calories—especially in the form of saturated fats. Saturated fats increase a dangerous form of blood cholesterol that is deposited like garbage in the walls of vital coronary arteries that supply blood to the rhythmically contracting heart muscle. If the blood supply to the heart is cut off, heart muscle cells die, and the heart itself may weaken or stop beating altogether. In some people, the narrowing of the coronary arteries occurs quietly without causing symptoms until the last moment (a heart attack). In others this narrowing leads to a form of chest pain upon exertion, called angina pectoris.

Of course, it's better to avoid this disease of our blood vessels entirely by taking preventive action. After all, we take good care of our automobiles and our homes, why not our own precious bodies? The answer is obvious when you think how easy it is to replace our possessions compared with trying to regain our lost health. Yet so often we take the extraordinary healing power of our bodies for granted and ignore risks that may take years to cause illness or even death. If you really want to reduce your risk of heart disease, follow the Lifelong Bran Plan, avoid smoking, exercise regularly, minimize stress and keep your weight at the level appropriate for your body frame and height.

Now you know that a diet low in fat, especially saturated fat, helps to prevent heart disease. And you've heard about the soluble fiber in oat bran helping to lower blood cholesterol, which in turn lowers the risk for heart disease because there is less cholesterol to clog up the arteries leading to the heart. In the 25 or more published studies showing the effect of oat bran on the cholesterol levels of humans, some showed a 23 percent reduction in cholesterol, others no change at all. However, the overwhelming weight of the research results clearly indicates that oat bran lowers cholesterol in both humans and animals. That's why we've included it in the Bran Cocktail (see page 31).

It's important to realize that a spoonful of oat bran a day will not lower your cholesterol level appreciably. The people in these studies consumed an ounce (⅓ cup dry or 1 cup cooked) to 5 ounces of bran daily. The more bran they were given, the greater the effect. Also, the higher the blood cholesterol level of the person, the more dramatic was the drop in cholesterol levels. For instance, among those in the study showing the greatest fall in cholesterol—23 percent—the average blood cholesterol level of the group was very high—309 mg/dl (over 200 is considered high). And they ate 3½ ounces of oat bran for three weeks.

The very characteristic that makes oatmeal and oat bran gummy and viscous is what causes the fall in cholesterol levels. According to the current theory on how these foods work, it all begins with the liver, where cholesterol is used to make bile acids (a kind of human detergent that helps to break up dietary fat so it's easier to absorb). The bile is stored in the gallbladder, to be released when a fat-containing meal comes rolling down the intestines. After the bile does its job, it is recycled back to the liver to be used again.

Here's where oat bran steps in. On its way down the intestines, the soluble fiber in oat bran absorbs water, expands, and forms a gel in the intestine. This mass of gel traps the bile so it can't go back to the liver, and the bile leaves the body as part of the stool. When the bile supply runs low, the liver draws upon the body's cholesterol stores to make new bile. That brings down the level of blood cholesterol, resulting in less damage to the arteries.

Other soluble fiber-rich brans also lower cholesterol, probably in the same manner. Psyllium seed, part of a grain grown primarily in India, has about eight times as much soluble fiber as oat bran, and studies show that it can lower cholesterol very effectively. In a University of

Kentucky study, men with an average cholesterol level of 250 mg/dl took one teaspoon of psyllium powder three times a day. After eight weeks the average cholesterol level fell by 14 percent. Psyllium is very potent and too much of it can cause bloating and other intestinal problems, so we've calculated a safe, effective amount of psyllium for the Bran Cocktail.

Rice bran (also part of the Bran Cocktail) works in another way. It's not particularly rich in soluble fiber, but rice bran is high in a special oil that helps to lower cholesterol even more effectively than the bran, although they probably act together. Rice bran oil contains more of the compounds called plant sterols than most oils do. These sterols look very much like cholesterol, and one theory holds that they may trick the body into recognizing them as cholesterol and allowing them to enter the body *in place of cholesterol.* (Since the number of sites where cholesterol can be absorbed into the system is limited, these sterols effectively block the cholesterol in many sites.)

Rice bran oil may lower cholesterol in yet another fashion. Again, it starts with the liver, which not only processes cholesterol from the diet and the bloodstream but also makes its own cholesterol. Researchers noticed that animals eating lots of rice bran or rice bran oil produced less cholesterol. They theorize that some compound in rice bran and its oil signals enzymes in the liver to reduce cholesterol production.

Barley research has just begun, but studies show that by consuming one cup of barley flour daily as cereal and in muffins, you can lower your cholesterol level by about 7 percent. Barley contains both soluble fiber and an oil similar to rice bran oil, so it may be influencing cholesterol levels in a number of ways.

Corn bran is another promising newcomer. In a study at Georgetown University School of Medicine, men with cholesterol levels above 240 mg/dl added about ½ ounce of corn bran to their daily diets for 6 weeks, then increased the level to 1¼ ounces for another 6 weeks. At the end of the entire 12-week period, they averaged a 20 percent drop in cholesterol levels. Study leader Jerry Earll, M.D., speculates that corn bran acts in a way similar to the cholesterol-lowering drug cholestyramine. Almost like oat bran, cholestyramine binds with bile acids, which are excreted instead of returned to the liver.

Too few studies have been done to allow us to recommend corn bran or barley at this time, however.

In addition to brans, certain fruits and vegetables are good sources of soluble fiber. Beans, or legumes, which include pinto beans, white beans, kidney beans, lentils, lima beans and chick-peas, are loaded with soluble fiber. Research shows that adding beans to the diet reduces blood cholesterol almost as effectively as oat bran.

In a University of Kentucky study, men with high cholesterol readings added ¾ cup of cooked beans to their daily diet. After 21 days, the average cholesterol level fell by 10 percent. We recommend beans because they are not only a good source of fiber but also an excellent source of protein, complex carbohydrates, certain B vitamins, iron and other minerals.

None of these foods will do much to protect you against heart disease if your staples are steak, premium ice cream and fettucine Alfredo. You must keep dietary fat intake down as well. Although some of the oat bran studies did show that oat bran can push cholesterol levels down a little bit in spite of a high-fat diet, the only really significant reduction in cholesterol levels came when oat bran was added to a low-fat diet. So you can see that all the bran that lowers cholesterol contains mostly soluble fiber. Wheat bran, while beneficial in other ways, has no effect on cholesterol whatsoever, because it is mostly insoluble fiber.

Strokes. A stroke occurs when a blood clot or some bleeding occurs in a diseased blood vessel in the brain. It can cause paralysis or weakness that usually affects only one side of the body. However, the stroke may also cause sight and speech problems. The greatest risk for a stroke is uncontrolled high blood pressure, but the same basic risk factors that increase your risk of heart disease also increase your risk of having a stroke. Again the advice is simple: Follow the basic low-fat/high-fiber dietary habits exemplified in the Lifelong Bran Plan—and avoid smoking!

Dietary Fiber Fights Cancer and Other Diseases

Several of our most deadly diseases are much less likely to occur in the presence of a high fiber intake. So we think it is very important that you don't miss out on such a simple means of protection.

Colon cancer and colonic polyps. Colon cancer is the second most common cause of death from cancer, affecting both sexes more or less equally. (Lung cancer caused by smoking is number one.) Fortunately, scientific literature strongly supports the belief that a diet low in fat and high in fiber, especially insoluble fiber like that found in whole grains and bran cereals, can significantly reduce the risk of cancer in various parts of the body, and especially in the colon. Comparison of groups of people in different countries and in different communities reveals that the more fiber you eat, the lower your risk of colon cancer. For example, New Yorkers who eat a lot of fat and little fiber were compared with people in Finland who also eat a lot of fat but much more fiber than New Yorkers. The results indicated that the high-fiber diet reduced colon cancer risk among the Finns. Another study revealed that Hispanics (who eat a diet high in cornmeal, beans, rice, peppers and other fiber-rich plant foods) in Los Angeles have at least a third fewer cases of colon cancer than residents of Connecticut, who have the highest rate of that disease in the nation and who eat a typical American diet.

A study of Seventh-Day Adventists, who eat a healthier high-fiber, low-fat diet that contains less meat than the typical American diet, compared their colon cancer rate with other American communities and found that their diet was protective. Some studies took a different approach, comparing the diets of those patients with colon cancer with the diets of the healthy population. These results are less convincing because often it is difficult to evaluate the influence of the disease itself on dietary habits.

As often happens in medicine, it is difficult to understand precisely why certain benefits occur. Some diseases can be successfully treated without the physician's knowing exactly how a drug worked, or sometimes why it worked at all. But in the case of fiber, the beneficial effects on the colon are known to be due to at least four factors.

First, the insoluble fiber that is a major part of wheat bran increases the bulk of the intestinal contents, not only speeding its travel time through the colon but also diluting the cancer-causing chemicals that are inevitably found there. This reduces the time the colon is exposed to these carcinogens, which reduces the risk.

Second, the insoluble fiber found in wheat bran also absorbs and removes some of the bile acids that are secreted as a result of stimulation by dietary fat. These bile acids, which normally help the body to digest and absorb fat, are also promoters of colon cancer. Anything that can reduce the amount of bile acids will therefore be helpful.

Third, the amount of fat absorbed in the presence of a high-fiber diet is almost certainly reduced in humans, since it was reduced in rats that were studied in our laboratory.

Fourth, there is evidence that stimulation of bacterial growth may help to neutralize the cancer-causing substances in the colon.

Nearly all cases of colon cancer arise in polyps (small mushroom-like growths) that have undergone a malignant change. These polyps are sometimes caused by an inherited genetic defect, but they far more often result from eating an unhealthy Western diet. Such polyps are extremely rare in developing countries where a low-fat, high-fiber diet is the norm.

In our own research laboratories at George Washington University Medical Center, we are studying the effects of various brans on colon cancer risk in laboratory animals. In some of these experiments, we gave the animals a diet high in fat and low in fiber, and compared their colon cancer risk to that of other groups of animals that received a bran-enriched version of the same diet. A substantial reduction in colon cancer risk showed up as a direct result of adding either wheat bran or psyllium. Other experiments presently under way will assess the effects of oat bran, rice bran and corn bran in this area.

A separate study demonstrated that animals fed a high-fat, low-fiber diet that was also low in calcium were in increased danger of developing colon cancer. When these same animals were switched to a healthy diet that was low in fat, high in calcium and high in bran fiber, their risk was dramatically reduced. The results of these animal experiments support the theory that people who have eaten *unhealthy* diets for years would benefit from switching to healthy diets. These very encouraging results have contributed greatly to our enthusiasm for promoting the adoption of the healthy Bran Plan diet by everyone.

Breast cancer. Cancer of the breast affects one in nine women, and it is second only to lung cancer as a cause of death from cancer in women. The good news is that many scientists believe the risk can be reduced by a change in eating habits. This is based on the fact that much evidence links breast cancer to a high intake of dietary fat in both laboratory animals and humans. Now some exciting studies at the

American Health Foundation in New York City have shown a remarkable reduction in breast cancer among rats that received a diet high in wheat bran, which is, of course, high in insoluble fiber. This benefit is credited to the reduced estrogen levels associated with a low-fat, high-fiber diet. For that reason as well as for its effects on colon cancer, wheat bran has been chosen as the major ingredient in the Bran Cocktail.

Diverticular disease and irritable colon (irritable bowel syndrome). A low-fiber diet also changes the normal functioning of the colon. One of the effects can be chronic constipation, which predisposes the colon to develop weaknesses in the wall, creating little pouches (diverticula) that can become infected or bleed. Another effect of a low-fiber diet is to encourage spasm of the muscles lining the wall of the colon (irritable colon) in those people who are susceptible to this condition.

Diverticular disease (diverticulosis) usually produces few symptoms unless some complication occurs: It is then called diverticulitis. Irritable colon is a condition often associated with anxiety, stress and intermittent constipation. In each of these conditions increased fiber intake should ease the symptoms and reduce the risk of complications.

Still More Bran Plan Benefits

Research shows that fiber also plays a role in preventing other ailments that can reduce your quality of life.

Hemorrhoids and varicose veins. Both these conditions involve distended veins and the possibility of painful symptoms caused by inflammation or phlebitis. Neither hemorrhoids nor varicose veins seem to occur in those countries where a high-fiber diet is customary. Since straining causes a tremendous increase in pressure within these veins, constipation is an obvious risk factor that can be avoided by consuming adequate dietary fiber. Another condition that predisposes women to these problems is pregnancy. This is because the enlarged uterus in some women may obstruct the flow of blood through the veins in the pelvis. The result is increased pressure that can distend the veins in the legs and pelvis and cause permanent dilatation, or stretching, of the vessel walls.

Diabetes. People in countries that follow a traditional diet high in fiber and complex carbohydrates rarely have diabetes, a disease that is so common in America partly because so many people are overweight. No one knows for sure whether changing to a high-fiber diet will lower your present risk of developing diabetes mellitus. But we do know that dietary fiber can play a major role in stabilizing diabetic patients. If you are one, you should discuss the value of added fiber with your personal physician.

Gallstones. The gallbladder is a small bag, which is just a few inches long, that is found underneath the liver. It stores bile produced in the liver and passes it to the intestine, especially in the presence of dietary fat. Typically, the patient who develops stones in the gall-bladder is "fair, fat, female and 40," although there are often exceptions to this description. It will come as no surprise that gallstones are rare among people in those countries where the traditional diets are low in fat and high in fiber. Surgical removal of gallstones often becomes necessary when they cause inflammation and unbearable pain. Following the Lifelong Bran Plan should reduce your risk of developing gallstones—a much more attractive choice than major abdominal surgery!

Obesity. Last, but not least, a high-fiber diet can help keep you trim. One reason is that you are so busy eating foods high in fiber, like whole grains and vegetables and fruits, that you don't eat fattening foods. Also, a high-fiber meal makes you feel full on fewer calories. And, if animal studies are a good indicator, fiber may "trap" some fat in the intestine so that less is absorbed—which means fewer calories!

Make Sure You Get All the Fiber You Need

An intense debate goes on among scientists about the amount of fiber it takes to provide optimal protection against disease and how much of each type of fiber we should eat. To settle these questions, expert committees of scientists were consulted by the National Cancer Institute and the Food and Drug Administration. The consensus was that the American diet should contain 20 to 35 grams of fiber per day. At present, the average American consumes 11 to 14 grams of fiber per day.

If your fiber intake is low, your first step should be to double your fiber intake by using the Bran Cocktail and by choosing more high-fiber foods. Even this amount is still much less than the fiber intake our bodies adapted to during thousands of years of evolution. It is also far lower than the 50 to 150 grams per day found in some African diets. But be assured, you will notice the difference. And you'll be on your way to the healthiest diet available that also helps control your weight.

So when you are planning meals or actually shopping for food, keep the fiber content of each food in mind. Learn to estimate approximately how much fiber your favorite foods and meals provide, so you can take greater control of your diet. (Appendix C on page 256 should help.) The Bran Plan was designed to make this a lot easier for you. Still, knowing all you can about what you're eating is very important if you are to control your food choices and weight, and be fit and healthy for life.

CHAPTER

3

Fat–A Deadly American Tradition

I t's as American as apple pie."
At 50 percent of calories from
fat, apple pie and other high-fat American staples have a lot to do with
a few other national traditions, like heart disease, cancer and obesity.
As noted in the previous chapter, by eating less than half of the recommended amount of fiber, Americans have set themselves up for a variety
of diseases. Likewise, eating double the healthy fat level contributes to
some of those same diseases as well as others. Before showing you how
to cut back on fat (chapters 9 and 10), we want to point out just how
dangerous (and fattening) a high-fat diet really is.

Dietary fat, especially when combined with smoking, is the single
most important cause of heart disease, and it's also a major cause of cancers of the breast, colon and prostate as well as the less common cancers that affect the ovaries, uterus and pancreas. Particularly sobering is
the fact that studies of children in the United States show that many of
them develop deposits of fatty cholesterol in the walls of their arteries
by the age of ten—a strong indication that they may develop heart dis-

---

ease in later life. And high-fat diets are a major reason that about one-third of Americans are overweight.

In the United States, the level of fat in the average diet adds up to nearly 40 percent—at least twice the optimum amount—of all the calories we eat. This means that those on the high end are taking in 70 percent or more of calories from fat, which could amount to several cups of fat each day. All this fat is coming from our meat-based diet, short on fiber-rich vegetables, whole grains and legumes and heavy on fried foods and fat-rich processed food products.

In countries with low levels of cancer and heart disease, one of the most striking observations is that the natives consume much less fat than we do. Recent studies in China, jointly conducted by Cornell University, the University of Oxford and Beijing University, show that lowering your fat intake means lowering your risk of cancer and heart disease—even down to a level of fat intake that is only 6 percent of total calories.

In Japan, where people live longer than anyplace else in the world, until recently fat in the diet accounted for only about 14 percent of calories. Their diet is becoming more Western, they are eating more fat and already their cancer and heart disease rates are on the rise. Even the Bran Plan's 20 percent of calories from fat still exceeds that found in some countries where the traditional diet is very low in fat. Keep this in mind when you hear that some official health organizations, for unscientific and political reasons, recommend reducing our fat intake to 30 percent of calories, which really is still far too much! Why aim for a level that is still associated with much cancer and heart disease in other countries? Surely it makes more sense to work toward a level of dietary fat that is *known* to reduce disease risk.

Of course, few of us know the exact amount of fat we eat, but this rough guide is helpful: If the average diet is 2,000 calories, then 20 percent (400 calories) from fat means you can eat 45 grams of fat per day. Since a teaspoon of fat or oil is equivalent to 5 grams of fat, you can see that we should limit ourselves to nine teaspoons per day. That's about half the amount of fat most Americans ordinarily eat. So to cover yourself, when in doubt, take half the usual portion of any food you know contains fat. Of course, it helps if you have taken the trouble to teach yourself where fat hides in your diet, and how to avoid it. The Lifelong Bran Plan (chapter 10) will show you how to keep your dietary fat intake low while hardly ever having to count fat grams.

Get a Fix on the Family of Fats

The fats in foods and fats in our bodies are called triglycerides. As you might expect, the chemical structure of triglycerides is made up of a "backbone" with *three* fatty acids attached. The main types of fatty acids are *saturated, monounsaturated* and *polyunsaturated,* and they have different chemical structures.

Any triglyceride may contain one or more types of these different fatty acids. Therefore, a triglyceride could be made up entirely of saturated fatty acids or a combination of saturated, monounsaturated and polyunsaturated fatty acids. Corn oil, for example, consists largely of polyunsaturated fatty acids but contains some saturated and monounsaturated fatty acids as well. In contrast, olive oil is made up mainly of monounsaturated fatty acids, with some saturated and polyunsaturated fatty acids included. This is important to understand because these fatty acids affect your body in very different ways.

Saturated fatty acids are the most harmful. They appear in animal products and in a few vegetable oils (coconut, palm and palm kernel), plus cocoa butter. Monounsaturated fatty acids and polyunsaturated fatty acids are less harmful, and they are found mostly in nuts and vegetable oils, such as canola, safflower, sunflower, corn, olive, soybean and cottonseed. On the other hand, cholesterol comes only from animal products and is often combined with fatty acids.

As a general rule, fats that are hard at room temperature, like lard and butter, are predominantly saturated; fats that are liquid at room temperature, like olive oil and peanut oil, are predominantly unsaturated. Both cholesterol and the triglycerides have an important influence on our risk of heart disease.

Finally, we have to consider the omega-3 fatty acids, a very important group of fats that are found mostly in fish. These fats seem to have the ability to lower cholesterol levels and actually reduce the risk of heart disease. In one study, for example, people who ate a diet rich in salmon for four weeks managed to reduce their blood cholesterol levels by 15 percent and their triglyceride levels by 38 percent (reducing cholesterol by 1 percent usually lowers heart disease risk by about 2 percent). In this study, the benefit was credited entirely to the presence of the omega-3 fatty acids. Cholesterol levels went down despite a salmon intake that provided about 500 milligrams of cholesterol each day, which had no obvious harmful effect although it is far above the already generous 300 milligrams a day recommended for heart health.

This study provides a good incentive for eating more fish and getting away from red meat, which is so high in cholesterol-raising saturated fat. Get your omega-3 from eating fish a couple of times a week, not from capsules. Capsules may "thin" the blood so that you may bleed too easily.

Dietary Fat Ends Up as Body Fat

No matter whether a fat is saturated or unsaturated, it has the same number of calories, and too much fat in any form puts you at risk for obesity. (See chapter 5 for more details.)

High-fat diets are usually high-calorie diets. At nine calories per gram, fat has more than double the calories of carbohydrate or protein. (Fiber, also a carbohydrate, has no calories.) An ounce of fat—peanut oil, for example, contains 256 calories, whereas an ounce of mostly carbohydrate (like cooked rice) or mostly protein (like skinless chicken breast) contains only about 40 calories.

Then there is another insidious fat fact: *It's a lot easier for your body to turn dietary fat into body fat than to convert carbohydrate or protein into fat.* That means, if you eat more calories than you need in the form of french fries or ice cream, that fat would sail right into your fat cells. But if your excess calories come from rice (carbohydrate), or skinless chicken, your body actually expends calories trying to turn them into fat. So, a high-fat diet will make you fatter than a low-fat diet, even if both diets contain the exact same number of calories.

Scientists have examined how women's weight fluctuates according to the amount of fat in their diets. One study, conducted in 1987, revealed that women who followed a low-fat diet spontaneously dropped their calorie intake by 11 percent. When they followed a high-fat diet, however, their calorie intake automatically increased by 15 percent. It's clear from this study that reducing fat intake really helps you cut your daily calorie consumption.

Aside from the social stigma of being overweight, it's usually unhealthy. Excess pounds can increase your risk for cancer, heart disease, high blood pressure, strokes, diabetes and joint or respiratory problems, among others. The good news is that at 20 percent of calories from fat, the Bran Plan for Weight Loss puts you at a healthy fat level (chapter 6).

Thin People Have Heart Attacks, Too

Even if you are not overweight, too much dietary fat is hard on your heart. The dietary fat that is not stored in your fat cells circulates in your blood as blood lipids (which consist of cholesterol and triglycerides). Saturated fat from your diet, much more than dietary cholesterol, raises the level of blood cholesterol. In fact, saturated fat increases blood cholesterol levels *four times* as much as cholesterol from your diet. Excess blood cholesterol can clog up the arteries leading to your heart. Eventually, your heart muscle can't get enough blood and oxygen; heart disease and heart attacks result.

People who eat low-fat diets have a much lower risk for heart disease, as many population studies have shown. Most notably, a fascinating study was conducted in Mexico among the Tarahumara Indians who live on the high plateaus of the Sierra Madre Mountains in the state of Chihuahua. The traditional foods of the Tarahumara over thousands of years have been corn and beans, some vegetables and fruits and small quantities of game, fish and eggs. Since their diet is very low in fat and cholesterol, it is not surprising that few of them ever develop coronary heart disease, and high blood pressure is virtually unknown. (Tarahumara means "fleet of foot," so you might guess that these people run a lot in their daily lives, which also helps to keep their cardiovascular systems in great shape.)

As part of this special study, a group of the Tarahumara was given a typical Western diet, like the one so many Americans eat—excessive in calories, high in fat, saturated fat and cholesterol and low in fiber. The effect was dramatic. Within five weeks, the levels of blood cholesterol in the Tarahumaras increased by more than 30 percent, their blood triglycerides went up by 18 percent and their average weight increased by 7 percent: just the sort of changes that usually indicate a significant increase in the risk of heart disease if such a diet is followed indefinitely. These experiments are a dramatic demonstration of the power diet has to change our bodies and to raise or lower our risk of disease. Yet again, we have evidence that the typical American diet is very unhealthful.

Nearly half of the two million deaths that occur each year in the United States are caused by cardiovascular diseases. Many of these deaths are caused by coronary heart disease, which is largely due to a narrowing of the coronary arteries that normally supply blood to the heart muscle. Diets high in saturated fats and cholesterol can lead to this dangerous narrowing, which can eventually result in a complete blockage, actually destroying the dependent heart muscle through lack of vital oxygen.

The main risk factors for coronary disease are high blood cholesterol, high blood pressure and smoking. Other less important risk factors are obesity, lack of exercise, short stature (taller people have fewer heart attacks), high triglyceride levels, stress, diabetes mellitus and a history of heart disease in the family. These risk factors also increase the risk for strokes, which are produced by the blockage of, or bleeding from, an artery in the brain.

We know that high cholesterol levels in the blood are mainly due to bad dietary habits, and we also know that high blood pressure rarely occurs in countries where the native diet is similar in balance to the Bran Plan. Among Americans who are overweight and eat too much salt (sodium), high blood pressure is quite common.

Cholesterol is carried in the blood by special proteins known as lipoproteins, which occur in two main types: high-density lipoproteins (HDL) and low-density lipoproteins (LDL). Think of these as the good cholesterol and the bad cholesterol, respectively. The basic difference is that HDL carries cholesterol away from the interior walls of arteries, while LDL deposits cholesterol in these walls.

Research has established that the ratio of HDL to LDL is an important way to predict heart disease risk. Further, the total amount of cholesterol and the total amount of HDL are also important indicators that can be monitored following dietary change or drug treatment.

How This Heart-Saver Diet Was Discovered

Until the seventeenth century, no one was aware of such a thing as arterial disease, and it took another 200 years to name it arteriosclerosis (hardening of the arteries). It was not until 1904 that researchers discovered fatty deposits clinging to the inner walls of arteries and called it *atherosclerosis*. Although a physician named J. B. Herrick, M.D., linked atherosclerosis to coronary heart disease in 1912, it took many years before it was widely recognized that atherosclerosis was a common cause of death. The first experiments linking diet and atherosclerosis were done on rabbits in 1908. A. I. Ignatovski, M.D., showed that rabbits fed a diet rich in meat, eggs and whole milk soon developed arterial disease similar to that seen in humans.

Soon after Dr. Herrick's announcement, other scientists identified cholesterol as the main dietary ingredient responsible for atherosclerosis in various types of animal species. Unfortunately, few scientists understood how these observations applied to human nutrition or to the rising number of deaths from heart disease. And, the bulk of the scientific community was ignorant of a 1916 report by a Dutch physician, C. D. DeLangen, M.D., that revealed native Indonesians had lower blood cholesterol levels and fewer cases of heart disease than Dutch colonists—until the Indonesians switched to a typical Dutch diet. Then their cholesterol levels and incidence of heart disease climbed dramatically. Written in Dutch and published in an obscure Dutch scientific journal, these critically important observations went unnoticed for 40 years!

Further reports associating fats, cholesterol and heart disease trickled in slowly. In 1934 and 1941, I. Snapper, M.D., reported on the low incidence of heart disease in China, which he attributed to low cholesterol consumption and minimal use of saturated fats. During World War II, when heart disease (and some cancers) declined throughout Europe, it was seen as the direct result of the scarcity of high-fat meat, eggs and dairy products. Not surprisingly, when prosperity returned after the war, so did the higher levels of heart disease and cancer!

In the 1940s and 1950s further studies reinforced the association between dietary fat, increased blood cholesterol and heart disease. Yet, some scientists remained skeptical. By the 1960s, experimental studies in humans demonstrated convincingly that dietary cholesterol did increase the level of blood cholesterol, although not as much as did saturated fats. Within the next decade researchers found that a diet dominated by *monounsaturated* fats, like the diet on the Greek island of Crete, where olive oil is the predominant fat, was associated with little heart disease and a long life expectancy. This is remarkable considering that this diet provides about 40 percent of calories from fat.

But only in the early 1990s did a carefully planned scientific study by Dean Ornish, M.D., of the University of California, San Francisco, demonstrate conclusively that a diet very low in fat and cholesterol, combined with exercise and stress control, could actually *reverse* heart disease by opening clogged arteries to improve the blood supply to the heart.

Along the same lines, Richard Peto of Oxford University analyzed about 20 studies in which dietary change or drugs were used to lower blood cholesterol. He found that, on average, the risk of heart disease fell by 16 percent if the cholesterol level was lowered by 10 percent. That sort of encouragement makes the effort to follow the low-fat, low-cholesterol, high-fiber Lifelong Bran Plan seem especially worthwhile.

Does Fat Affect Your Blood Pressure?

When it comes to the role of fat in high blood pressure, the research is less conclusive. Although, in many cases, the cause of high blood pressure is unknown, it is well established that the problem occurs more often among Americans who are overweight, exercise little or have a low calcium intake, and less frequently among vegetarians. Although excessive salt intake has been associated with an increased risk of hypertension, there is no evidence that vegetarians consume less salt than nonvegetarians. The simple reason for their lower risk of hypertension may be that vegetarians prefer foods containing mono- and polyunsaturated fatty acids and eat less fat and cholesterol. However, few if any scientific studies have actually demonstrated that total fat intake influences the risk of hypertension.

One particularly interesting study compared Benedictine monks with Trappist monks and revealed that hypertension occurred in 51 percent of the Benedictines and in only 12 percent of Trappists. Both groups ate similar diets, with no difference in total fat intake. However, the healthier Trappists consumed relatively more vegetable fat, which means more monounsaturated and polyunsaturated fatty acids such as those found in olive oil and canola oil.

Some research has demonstrated a modest reduction in blood pressure when people switched from a typical high-fat diet to a low-fat diet similar to the one we recommend in the Bran Plan. A diet that is low in salt, cholesterol, saturated fat and total fat will not only protect your arteries but could also minimize your risk of developing hypertension.

Exciting News about Cancer Protection

Of all the elements in food that can increase your cancer risk, none is more important than fat. Numerous international studies reveal a strong association between the amount of dietary fat and the risk of developing cancer of the breast, colon, rectum, prostate and endometrium, and to a lesser extent, cancers of the kidney, ovaries and testicles.

Scientists studying the risk of breast cancer among women in different countries, have often seen large differences in the frequency with which it occurs. In Japan, for example, breast cancer is rare, while in the United States it is quite common, occurring in about one in nine women. When Japanese women migrated to the United States years ago, their breast cancer risk went up considerably, so that it became comparable to that of American women within about two generations. This observation was very significant because it meant that the risk of breast cancer was primarily tied to environmental factors, not genetic ones. And of all the environmental factors, dietary fat was found to be the most important. In a sense this is good news. If cancer was mostly genetic or inherited, we could do little about it. However, since about a third of our cancer risk is due to bad dietary habits and another third is due to smoking, adopting a healthy, low-fat, high-fiber diet will significantly reduce the risk of some cancers.

As early as the 1940s, researchers demonstrated that high levels of dietary fat could increase breast cancer risk in laboratory animals. Since then, many published studies have confirmed the relationship between dietary fat and breast cancer. However, a recent study of 80,000 nurses shows that the women who consumed 38 percent of their calories from fat had a greater risk of colon cancer, but their risk of breast cancer was no different than those whose intake of fat was 29 percent of total calories. The probable explanation: Steadily reducing fat intake reduces colon cancer risk, while the risk of breast cancer drops only when the fat intake is far less than 29 percent. Many experts believe that benefits begin to kick in only when the diet contains 20 percent or fewer total calories from fat. Incidentally, studies have also demonstrated that wheat bran can reduce the risk of breast cancer and colon cancer in laboratory rats, even if those rats were fed high-fat diets. These animal experiments support human studies that suggest a link between high-fat diets and cancer risk.

Colon and rectal cancer occurs more or less equally in men and women and is the second most common cancer, next to prostate cancer in men and breast cancer in women.

Of course, many studies of colorectal cancer have suggested a link with dietary fat. A major study that compared the diet of low-risk Finns in the town of Kuopio with that of high-risk Danes in the city of Copenhagen showed that although the fat intake of both groups was about the same, the fiber intake was much higher in the low-risk group. A study published in 1991 examined the dietary habits of thousands of nurses and found that those nurses who regularly ate red meat, which is high in fat, had a substantial increase in the risk of colon cancer.

Similarly, many studies tie prostate cancer to a high-fat diet. The latest figures indicate that this cancer affects more than 130,000 men annually in the United States. In Japan prostate cancer is rare, but in those parts of Japan where the diet is becoming Westernized (higher in fat), the incidence of this cancer is rising.

Most of the evidence derived from comparing the risks in different groups of people, often in different countries, suggests that the total fat in the diet is what counts. The degree of risk may depend on specific fats, however. For example, the omega-3 fatty acids found in fish may actually inhibit cancer formation, and monounsaturated fats like those abundant in olive oil are more or less neutral in their effects on cancer risk.

The study in China mentioned earlier confirmed the importance of dietary fat levels in relation to the risk of developing cardiovascular disease and cancer. At each level of dietary fat the researchers looked at—from 6 percent of calories to 40 percent of calories—they found that the higher the fat intake among the people studied, the greater the risk of developing cancer and heart disease. So, when we say that the level of fat in your diet is so important, believe us, it is!

The Bran Plan makes it easier than ever before to switch to a low-fat diet. Follow the Bran Plan for Weight Loss (chapter 6) and you'll be taking in no more than 20 percent of calories from fat. Because you'll be eating real food like fajitas and bagels, you'll hardly notice the drop in fat. The Lifelong Bran Plan (chapter 10) lets you work down to a healthy fat level at your own pace, one food group at a time. Using the Bran Cocktail (page 31) leaves you feeling full and satisfied on fewer calories, so you really won't miss the fat.

4

Your First Week on the Bran Plan

*N*ow is the time to begin to change the way you eat, the way you feel and, ultimately, the way you look—perhaps forever. You are about to start the one-week transition that will help you to leave some of your old eating habits behind and begin the process of replacing them with new patterns that will become a fundamental part of your life over the next few weeks, months and years.

New habits take time to become ingrained. Old habits were acquired over a lifetime, so expect it to take at least a month or more before you can succeed in making some permanent changes in your dietary habits. In the beginning, eating right takes planning. Later you'll find that it has become automatic. That's the easiest diet plan of all.

To help you, we've created a transition week that will introduce your body and your mind to the Bran Plan. It will eliminate that "overnight" psychological shock that we all instinctively rebel against when change occurs too suddenly. Also, this week will give your body a chance to get used to a higher-fiber diet, since both the Bran Plan for Weight Loss and the Lifelong Bran Plan will provide your body with much more disease-preventing fiber than it probably has been accustomed to.

Remember, follow this introductory plan *before* you start the Bran Plan for Weight Loss or the Lifelong Bran Plan. It'll be painless—instead of cutting foods out of your regular diet, you'll simply *add* two foods and our special Bran Cocktail each day. Nothing that will make you gain weight, just foods that will increase your fiber intake and get you used to eating something healthy.

After this week, if you want to lose weight, you can move on to the Bran Plan for Weight Loss in chapter 6. If you don't need to lose weight but want to eat in the healthiest way to protect yourself against disease for the rest of your life, you can go to the Lifelong Bran Plan in chapter 10.

It is very important for you to understand that you can go back and forth between the weight-loss plan and the lifelong eating plan. For instance, if the holidays have left you with a few excess pounds, you can slip into the Bran Plan for Weight Loss for a few weeks. Since the weight-loss plan is not excessively low in calories, going on and off it won't get you into the dangerous yo-yo cycle of weight swings, which slows down metabolism, making it even harder to lose weight.

The Bran Cocktail

Your first week of the Bran Plan is simple: *All you have to do is add the Bran Cocktail, one fruit and one vegetable serving to your diet each day.* Your score on the fiber quiz (page 32) will determine the amount of Bran Cocktail you should take.

The Bran Cocktail is not a drink—it's our special blend of four brans that will give you a carefully designed balance of fibers. This formula is based on a ratio of one part rice bran, two parts psyllium, four parts oat bran and eight parts wheat bran—proportions developed from an analysis of many scientific studies on fiber and health (see chapter 2 for details).

In addition to the Bran Cocktail, the extra fruit and vegetable servings will also contribute fiber and give you an extra measure of vitamins, minerals and other health-protecting nutrients.

Bran Cocktail

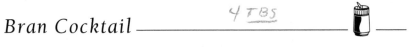

4 TBS

½ cup rice bran	2 cups oat bran
1 cup powdered psyllium	4 cups wheat bran

Combine the rice bran, psyllium, oat bran and wheat bran in a large mixing bowl. Transfer the mixture to a wide-mouthed jar or other airtight container, like Tupperware or Rubbermaid, and store it in a cool spot or in the refrigerator; heat can spoil stored brans.

Makes 7½ cups
5 grams dietary fiber per 2-tablespoon serving

Where to find the ingredients: Rice bran is sometimes in the "dietetic" section of supermarkets. If you can't find it there, you can order it from Ener-G Foods, P.O. Box 84487, Seattle, WA 98124-5787; 1-800-331-5222 or, in Washington, 1-800-325-9788. If you can't find it, skip it. The formula will still be effective, although not as perfectly balanced.

Psyllium is sold in most health food stores. Get the powdered type—the raw husks are too tough on the intestines. If you have trouble getting pure psyllium, go with unflavored Metamucil or another bulk-forming laxative that contains psyllium as the primary ingredient. This is available at drugstores. If you're using something other than Metamucil, ask the pharmacist to confirm that it's psyllium.

Oat bran and wheat bran are usually sold in supermarkets, in the hot cereal section or with baking ingredients. They are also available in health food stores. If you can't find wheat bran, substitute the same amount of Kellogg's All-Bran (Extra Fiber) cereal; lightly pulverize the All-Bran by running it through your blender for three seconds, or by crushing it with the back of a spoon.

To find out how much Bran Cocktail to add to your diet and to discover how your current fiber intake measures up to the recommended levels, take the fiber quiz on page 32. Tally your score, then look at the Bran Cocktail Prescription that accompanies each score to see how much cocktail to add to your diet. Later, we'll show you how to add it.

How Much Fiber Are You Getting?

The National Cancer Institute recommends eating 20 to 35 grams of fiber daily. This is the level that many researchers now believe helps protect us from some types of cancer and even heart disease by helping to lower cholesterol. (See chapter 2 to learn how fiber may help you live longer by protecting you from killer diseases.) Most Americans take in less than a third of that. This quiz will show you how your fiber intake compares with the recommended levels, but it will only provide you with an estimate of your actual intake; don't worry if you cannot answer the questions exactly. After you've been on the Bran Plan for a while, you can take the quiz again to measure your improvement.

Your Fiber Intake Quiz

Circle the number of points that corresponds most closely to your intake of the following foods.

Food	How Often?	Points
1. Two slices of whole grain bread (whole wheat, whole wheat plus oat bran or other whole grain bread) or 4 rye or whole wheat crackers	daily	8
	5 days/wk.	6
	3 days/wk.	(3)
	1 day/wk.	1
	never	0
2. One bowl of high-fiber bran cereal such as Kellogg's All-Bran or equivalent (check package label—1 serving should contain 9 grams or more of dietary fiber)	daily	24
	5 days/wk.	17
	3 days/wk.	10
	1 day/wk.	(1)
	never	0
3. One bowl of whole grain or bran cereal such as raisin bran, Fiberwise or Nutri-Grain (check package label— 1 serving should contain at least 3 grams of dietary fiber)	daily	9
	5 days/wk.	6
	3 days/wk.	(4)
	1 day/wk.	1
	never	0
4. One bowl of any of these hot cereals: oatmeal or oat bran, whole wheat, mixed grain or other whole grains	daily	8
	5 days/wk.	6
	3 days/wk.	(3)
	1 day/wk.	1
	never	0

Food	How Often?	Points
X **5.** One bran muffin	daily	5
	5 days/wk.	4
	3 days/wk.	2
	1 day/wk.	1
	never	0
X **6.** One cup of whole wheat pasta, brown rice or Kashi cereal	daily	11
	5 days/wk.	8
	3 days/wk.	5
	1 day/wk.	2
	never	0
X **7.** Any of the following: 3 apricots, ¼ cantaloupe, 1 peach, ½ cup pineapple, 5 plums, 3 dates or 1 cup watermelon	daily	4
	5 days/wk.	3
	3 days/wk.	2
	1 day/wk.	1
	never	0
8. Any of the following: 1 apple, banana or pear; 3 prunes; ¼ cup raisins; ½ cup raspberries or 1 cup strawberries	daily	6
	5 days/wk.	4
	3 days/wk.	③
	1 day/wk.	1
	never	0
9. One cup raw or ½ cup cooked of the following vegetables: asparagus, bean sprouts, cauliflower, celery, green peppers, kale, mushrooms, red or white cabbage, spinach, string beans, tomatoes, turnips or zucchini, or 1 medium potato without skin or ½ sweet potato	daily	4
	5 days/wk.	3
	3 days/wk.	②
	1 day/wk.	1
	never	0
10. One-half cup cooked of the following vegetables: broccoli, brussels sprouts, corn or parsnips, or 1 medium potato with skin	daily	6
	5 days/wk.	4
	3 days/wk.	3
	1 day/wk.	①
	never	0

Food	How Often?	Points
11. One-half cup of legumes (cooked dried beans) such as chick-peas, dried peas, lima beans or lentils, or fresh green peas	daily 5 days/wk. 3 days/wk. 1 day/wk. never	8 6 3 ① 0
12. One-half cup of the following cooked legumes: baked beans, kidney beans or navy beans	daily 5 days/wk. 3 days/wk. 1 day/wk. never	15 11 6 2 0

SCORING

Add up your circled points, then follow the Bran Cocktail Prescription that matches your score, below.

1 to 12 points—very low fiber level: At less than six grams of fiber per day, your diet is very low in fiber. This may put you at increased risk for colon cancer, constipation, appendicitis, gallstones, varicose veins and diverticulitis (an intestinal disease); and perhaps for diabetes, heart disease and obesity as well.

The Bran Cocktail Prescription: For the first two days, take three tablespoons of Bran Cocktail each day, which will add about seven grams of fiber to your diet. Then, if you are experiencing no intestinal discomfort (diarrhea, excessive gas), increase the Bran Cocktail to six tablespoons per day (15 grams of fiber).

13 to 22 points—low fiber level: Your diet is still low in fiber, in the range of 6.5 to 11 grams per day. More fiber would put you at less risk for diseases of the bowel, including colon and rectal cancer.

The Bran Cocktail Prescription: Add four tablespoons of Bran Cocktail to your diet each day, which will add about ten grams of fiber.

23 to 40 points—average American fiber level: At 11.5 to 20 grams of fiber daily, you're taking in more fiber than many Americans, but more would help you control your dietary balance and give you extra protection against diseases of the bowel, including colon and rectal cancer.

The Bran Cocktail Prescription: Add three tablespoons of Bran Cocktail to your diet daily. This will add about seven grams of fiber.

40-plus points—desirable fiber level: At about 20 grams of fiber per day, your fiber level is just adequate. You are already doing a lot to protect yourself from cancer, coronary heart disease and diseases of the bowel, but would still benefit from an increase.

The Bran Cocktail Prescription: If you'd like to ensure a well-rounded blend of the various types of fiber, add two tablespoons of the Bran Cocktail each day.

Periodically, you should do this test again and adjust your intake of the Bran Cocktail according to your new fiber quiz score.

Now here's a special tip: *It's crucial that you drink at least two extra 8-ounce glasses of water every day while adding the Bran Cocktail.*

One of the ways bran helps make you feel full and traps potential carcinogens is by absorbing water and swelling up in your gut. If you don't drink enough water, you may actually become constipated, because the swollen bran can't move quickly through your system. So drink at least two more glasses of water, or even more if you feel like it, each day *in addition to* what you normally drink.

How to Add the Bran Cocktail to Your Diet

Once you've made up a batch of Bran Cocktail in, say, a six-cup Rubbermaid plastic container, you might find it easier to transfer your daily allowance from the larger container into either a smaller ½-cup Rubbermaid container or a shaker, preferably one with large holes.

What we found also works well is an empty Parmesan cheese, paprika, parsley or oregano container (the kind with a slot for pouring or holes for shaking). You can even make your own shaker by punching holes in the top of an empty coffee tin or oatmeal container. It's okay to leave this small amount out on the kitchen table, but remember to keep the larger batch in a cool place. You can also keep a shaker in your office or wherever you wind up eating your meals. Replenish your small portable container as needed.

We've found that the Bran Cocktail blends in especially well with certain foods, such as cereal, cooked grains, stews and yogurt shakes to

Some Foods That Go with the Bran Cocktail

Applesauce

Bean dishes (such as chili or baked beans)

Burritos with any filling

Cereals (both hot and cold)

Green salads (add a little to the low-fat dressing)

Ground turkey or lean beef burgers (see "Cooking with the Bran Cocktail"

Indian curry

Mashed potatoes (made with skim milk and no fat)

Muffins and fruit breads (such as banana bread)

Pancakes

Pasta with tomato sauce and most other sauces

Pasta salads

Rice and other cooked grains

Most soups, especially lentil, thick minestrone, and other thick types

Stews

Tuna or chicken salad

Vegetable stir-fries

Yogurt (low-fat and nonfat)

Yogurt fruit shakes (low-fat and nonfat)

name a few. We've given you some suggestions above, and we've marked certain dishes in the menus in chapter 7 with the symbol indicating that they can easily be supplemented with the Bran Cocktail. You'll probably discover other ways to add the brans.

Don't think you have to shake the Bran Cocktail onto every food. It really doesn't go very well with broiled fish, most meats or certain delicate preparations. You can add a whole tablespoon or more of the brans to foods that mix well with it, such as cereal, stews, curries and chili, while just a teaspoon or two will suffice in soups and other dishes.

Experiment to see how much you can add to various foods without sacrificing flavor. Cooking with the brans will make rice and muffins taste even better, giving them a wonderful texture and a richer flavor.

You don't have to shake the entire day's Bran Cocktail prescription on one food. If, for instance, you are using two tablespoons of Bran Cocktail daily, you could sprinkle one tablespoon on your morning cereal, add ½ tablespoon to your lunch salad, and mix the final ½ tablespoon with your rice or pasta at dinner.

Cooking with the Bran Cocktail

If you cook rice or other grains with the Bran Cocktail, you should add more water than usual. For instance, if you add ¼ cup of Bran Cocktail to 1 cup of uncooked rice, add an extra ½ cup of water to the amount you usually use to cook the rice.

If you mix Bran Cocktail into pancakes or other batters, remember to add enough to make each serving bran-rich. For instance, if your recipe makes 12 muffins and you want each serving to contain a tablespoon of Bran Cocktail, you need to add 12 tablespoons (¾ cup) of the cocktail to the batter (see below).

Cooking Conversion Chart

If recipe calls for	Reduce to	Add this much Bran Cocktail	Add this much more liquid (milk, water, etc. depending on recipe)
2 cups flour	1¼ cups	¾ cup	3 Tbsp.
1½ cups flour	1 cup	½ cup	⅛ cup
1 cup flour	¾ cup	¼ cup	1 Tbsp.
1 cup grains (barley, bulgur, millet, polenta, rice, etc.)	no change	⅓ cup ¼ cup	⅔ cup ½ cup

Believe it or not, the Bran Cocktail works well in low-fat meat or turkey burgers (ask you butcher to grind the low-fat cuts of meat listed in appendix B on page 205). Simply soak the bran in an equal amount of water for two minutes. Drain off the excess water. Then mix the Bran Cocktail with the meat in a ratio of one part bran to three parts meat. For example, use ½ cup soaked bran to 1½ cups ground meat.

An Apple a Day...

Whether you scored high or low in our fiber quiz, you must add a serving of fruit and a vegetable serving to your diet each day of week one. Not only will this give you some extra fiber and vitamins and minerals, it will also get you into the habit of doing something healthy for your diet each day. During your first week, choose any fruits or vegetables you like, except avocados, which are quite high in fat and calories.

Fruits should be eaten raw and plain. Buy what's in season and most appealing. See page 158 for a list of some possible choices.

Vegetables should be raw, steamed, boiled or *very lightly* stir-fried in a minimum of oil. (French fries or other deep-fried vegetables don't count—they're saturated with oil.) If you eat your extra vegetable serving in the form of a salad, don't smother it with dressing. Potatoes and other starchy vegetables are higher in calories and are closer to breads and grains, so we've put them in a different food category (see chapter 10). When we ask you to add one vegetable to your daily diet, add at least 1 cup raw or ½ cup cooked. See page 159 for some suggestions about vegetable choices.

Have a wonderful, healthy week!

5

Are You Overweight– And Why?

*F*at: On our bodies it's the bane of our existence; in cheesecake and burgers, it's one of our greatest pleasures. But whatever the form, too much fat can *kill*, by contributing to heart disease, cancer and other deadly diseases. Despite this danger, fat consumption by Americans is among the highest in the world, constituting nearly 40 percent of our total calories. In poorer countries around the world that we think suffer so many disadvantages, people typically consume only about 10 percent of total calories as fat and only rarely experience heart disease and cancer—diseases that cause the majority of premature deaths among Americans.

In this chapter you'll get to know the enemy, find out why it settles on a woman's thighs (when she'd rather it go to her breasts) and why men find it harder with each passing year to stave off a belly. If you're carrying around extra fat, this chapter will be especially helpful, because once you start to understand *why* you're overweight, you can start to effectively do something about it. And there's new research giving us more ammunition than ever to fight the battle of the bulge.

There are only a few foods that are nearly 100 percent fat—lard, butter, margarine, chicken or bacon fat (or other meat drippings) and vegetable and grain oils. Some foods are high in fat but also contain some carbohydrate and protein. An example is the peanut, which is 50 percent fat by weight, 29 percent protein and 20 percent carbohydrate. (That's by weight; in terms of calories, 76 percent comes from fat.)

Fat According to Whom?

Experts are still groping for a standard definition of obesity. The new thinking is that how *much* you weigh is much less important than *where* on the body you carry the weight. Further on in this chapter you'll learn why having a big belly is more harmful to your health than carrying the fat in your hips and thighs.

For now, the best way to determine if you are unhealthfully heavy is to figure out your waist-to-hip ratio. With a measuring tape, measure around your midsection at the navel, as you stand relaxed (not sucking in your stomach). Then measure around the buttocks where they are the largest to get your hip measurement. Divide the waist measurement by the hip measurement to get your waist-to-hip ratio. Women with a ratio of 0.85 or above, and men with a ratio of 0.95 or above, may be at risk for some of the diseases associated with being overweight or obese. Read on to find out why this ratio is unhealthy and what you can do to bring it down to a healthy number.

Why Do We Get Fat?

The reason people get fat is both very simple and complicated enough to fuel research teams the world over. Simply, it's because a person eats more calories than he or she burns, and the excess is stored as fat. These calories could come from protein, carbohydrate or fat, but fat is more often the culprit because it has more than twice the calories of these other two macronutrients. That means, in theory, you could get fat from eating too much fruit (carbohydrate) or too much skinless chicken breast (protein), but no one does. It's the fat/carbohydrate mixtures (ice cream) or fat/protein mixtures (hamburger) or just plain fat (butter) that really stick it to you.

So there is a simple fact that you must know: You will gain weight if you eat more calories than your body needs. But why some people are able to burn more excess calories and others store those calories as fat is not always clear, although obesity experts are now able to make more accurate diagnoses.

Were You Born to Be Fat?

It used to be thought that people were fat either because they lacked willpower or inherited bad genes. Genes are minute blueprints found in every one of your cells that determine every physical aspect of you—the color of your eyes and hair, your height, whether you'll form the enzyme that digests milk sugar, and so forth. Now obesity experts know that while genes *are* a factor in determining body weight, whether you'll become fat depends on a complex interaction between genetics and lifestyle.

The best clue to discovering your genetic tendencies for obesity is to look at your parents. A child with parents who are not overweight has less than a 20 percent chance of becoming overweight. The chances increase to 40 percent with one obese parent and 80 percent when both parents are overweight. Some of the influence on weight may be environmental—the child picks up bad eating and exercise habits from Mommy and Daddy—but studies with adopted children indicate a strong genetic influence.

To separate the genetic influences from the lifestyle influences on obesity, researchers have compared adopted children to their biological and adoptive parents. One such study at the University of Pennsylvania divided 540 adult adoptees into four weight classes—thin, average weight, overweight and obese—and compared the adoptees' weight to that of their biological parents and their adoptive parents. The results indicated that the weight of the adult adoptees was very strongly related to that of their biological parents and *not at all to that of their adoptive parents*. So, an adopted boy whose biological parents were thin would probably end up thin, even if his adoptive parents were fat.

This and other studies show that your weight *is* strongly influenced by genetics, that you inherit the tendency to be fat, average or thin. But just because you've inherited the tendency doesn't mean it can't be controlled, as we'll show you later.

How Do Your Genes Make You Fat?

The genetic forces that conspired to make you fat may be different from the ones that have made your neighbor fat. Although obesity researchers have not yet pinpointed exactly which genes contribute to making people fat, they know some of the different effects of genes. For instance, your genes may be responsible for a slower metabolism or for directing fat to your hips and thighs, whereas your friend's genes send the fat to his stomach.

A fascinating study at Laval University in Quebec, using sets of identical twins, shows the genetic variation in weight gain. Researchers gave 12 pairs of male identical twins the same diet, letting calories vary according to the level where each man maintained his body weight, neither gaining nor losing. Then, on top of this base diet, they gave each man an extra 1,000 calories for 6 days a week for 100 days. As you might have predicted, with each set of identical twins, each twin gained the same amount of weight. But there was another result of this study that was even more revealing about the strong influence of genetics on weight gain—that was the striking *difference* in weight gain among different sets of identical twins. The average weight gain among all sets of identical twins was about 18 pounds, but look at the extremes: One set of twins gained only 10 pounds each, while another set gained 29 pounds each. And they were all getting the same amount of exercise.

There are many different genetic reasons why one set of twins may gain more weight than another, just as there are many different genetic reasons that make some people fatter than others.

One of these genetically influenced factors is metabolic rate—the rate at which a person burns calories. A person with a "slow" metabolism burns fewer calories than most people. Genetics can influence the rate at which calories are burned at rest (lying down, sitting still or sleeping). Genetics also influence the amount of calories it takes to digest a meal and the calories expended during exercise. That means one man on a rowing machine might burn only 70 percent as many calories as the man on the rowing machine next to him, even if both men are exercising with equal vigor and are of the same height and build. How genes can slow your metabolism is still unclear.

Interestingly, your genes may even regulate *how much* you exercise. In a Massachusetts Institute of Technology study comparing infants born to obese and normal-weight mothers, half of the infants born to obese mothers became overweight by the time they'd reached one year of age. The overweight infants ate the same amount and type of food as the normal-weight infants and had similar resting metabolic rates. But overweight infants were less active than others. The researchers speculate that the overweight infants were simply imitating inactive siblings or parents, or that their relative inactivity had a genetic origin. The results of this study prompted the researchers to suggest that parents should increase the exercise level of their obese infants instead of restricting their food, which could put them at risk for nutritional deficiencies.

Does Your Sex Make a Difference?

Women are naturally fatter than men, even though newborn males and females start out the same, with fat constituting about 12 percent of body weight at birth—fatter than any other newborn mammal except the whale. Lacking a protective layer of fur, we need that fat to keep us warm. During puberty, girls get fatter and boys get leaner. By age 18, girls have 20 to 25 percent body fat and most boys have 15 to 18 percent. Adults steadily put on weight, so by middle age, fat constitutes about 30 to 40 percent of body weight for both sexes. But women still retain a slight edge. Women evolved with extra body fat mainly to provide a reserve of calories, which is especially important during pregnancy and breastfeeding.

Fat also settles differently on men and women. Men's fat usually goes straight to their bellies, women's to their hips and thighs. One way of classifying obesity is by shape. Apple-shaped people, with a large waist-to-hip ratio, carry much of their extra body fat in their bellies and are at increased risk for heart disease and diabetes and have lower levels of HDLs—the "good" cholesterol carrier. It's still not clear exactly why abdominal fat is so risky, but one hypothesis is that unlike hip and thigh fat, which stays put, abdominal fat is constantly flowing in and out of fat cells, creating more circulating blood fat that can clog up the arteries and cause heart disease. Those with pear shapes, even if obese, are not at increased risk. As we mentioned at the beginning of this chapter, certain waist-to-hip ratios are considered risky. "*Where* the fat settles is much more important than *how much* fat you have," says noted obesity research scholar Jean-Pierre Després, Ph.D., of Laval University. "I can't emphasize enough that two obese people with the same amount of body fat may have very different health risks," he adds.

Have you ever wondered why even fairly athletic men can't seem to avoid a belly? "Testosterone, the main male hormone, seems to help remove fat from abdominal cells," says Marielle Rebuffé-Scrive, Ph.D., a biochemist and associate professor at Yale University. As men age, their testosterone levels decrease, so a 50-year-old will have more trouble burning fat than a 20-year-old, she explains. With age, the risk of accumulating more abdominal fat and becoming apple-shaped increases. In one of her research studies, she gave middle-aged men a dose of testosterone, which increased the removal of body fat from abdominal fat cells. She's currently studying the effects of long-term testosterone supplementation to see whether it truly helps men get rid of their spare tires.

Hormones affect the way fat is deposited in women as well. Women can thank the female hormones estrogen and progesterone for fat that gravitates to the hip and thigh region. During pregnancy, women accumulate even more lower-body fat as a reserve to be used in breastfeeding. Breastfeeding burns an extra 800 daily calories. Dr. Rebuffé-Scrive's studies indicate that hip and thigh fat is the most difficult to lose because women's hormones and enzymes favor depositing, not removing, fat in that region—except during breastfeeding, which switches off the fat-storing enzyme, lipoprotein lipase. This allows hip and thigh fat to be converted to energy to fuel milk production in the breasts.

After menopause, levels of female hormones fall, and if women aren't careful, they will start accumulating fat in a more malelike pattern—in the belly. The extra abdominal fat is one factor putting women at the same increased risk as men for heart disease. In other words, a changing distribution of body fat is a sign that the arteries supplying blood to the heart may also be deteriorating. "As women go beyond menopause, they develop higher cholesterol levels than men—20 to 30 percent higher," according to Michael DeBakey, M.D., chairman of the Department of Surgery at Baylor College of Medicine in Texas, who operates on quite a few postmenopausal women with heart disease. Recent studies suggest that fat concentrated in the abdominal area also places women at increased risk for breast cancer.

But even before they reach menopause, 22 percent of obese women are apple-shaped, according to studies at the Medical College of Wisconsin. These women are at increased risk for heart disease and diabetes, just like the men and postmenopausal women with excess belly fat.

Again, hormones are the culprit. Men and women have both male and female sex hormones. Apple-shaped premenopausal women just have slightly less female hormones (and slightly more male hormones) than other women. The altered hormonal levels are so slight that no one would ever notice, but these women are predisposed to accumulate more belly fat.

What Else Is Making You Fat?

Even if both your parents are fat, and even if scientists pinpointed the exact sets of genes that contribute to obesity, and even if you had them all, you might still prevent the problem. Because unlike the eye color you inherited, you *can do something* about the tendency for obesity. It's just a harder task for someone with "fat genes" than for someone with "thin genes." Even if you're genetically predisposed, you can ward off excess fat if you keep calories under control and increase exercise. But to really carve away at body fat, it's often not enough simply to reduce calories—you must make sure that a smaller percentage of those calories come from fat. A study by the U.S. Department of Agriculture's Agricultural Research Service has shown that women can slightly reduce body fat by switching from 40 percent to 20 percent of total calories from fat even *without lowering their normal daily calorie level.*

The reason low-fat diets help is that it's harder to get fat by eating protein and carbohydrate. Turning carbohydrate and protein into stored fat is hard work for the body, but excess dietary fat has an easy route into your fat cells. Both the Bran Plan for Weight Loss and the Lifelong Bran Plan are low in fat so that you will shed body fat, not accumulate it.

Besides the fat level of your diet, there's another dietary habit that may make a difference—alcohol. Studies in Italy and Sweden show that women who drink more alcohol and/or smoke tend to be more apple-shaped. Why? One hypothesis: A high intake of alcohol may create slightly higher levels of male hormones, which means fat is deposited in the abdomen instead of in the hips and thighs.

Dieting, especially yo-yo dieting (periods of low-calorie dieting followed by periods of overeating) may also affect body shape. Research at the University of California, Davis, found that with every yo-yo cycle, rats tended to accumulate more fat in the abdominal area. A veteran dieter who has been dieting for the past ten years could easily have gone through 30 or more yo-yo cycles.

The Bran Plan avoids the yo-yo syndrome by never dipping below 1,200 calories, which is a good, safe calorie level for most moderately active women. It also provides two other higher calorie levels for men and very active women.

Is It Ever Okay to Be Fat?

Research has shown that being mildly obese seems to actually be healthier once you get older. A Johns Hopkins University School of Medicine study found that with the exception of 55- to 64-year-old women, thin 55- to 75-year-olds of both sexes died earlier than those 20 to 30 percent over "ideal" body weight. Researchers suspect that the thinner people died earlier because they were suffering from malnutrition, especially inadequate amounts of calories and protein, which may have weakened their immune systems. As you get older, it's more important to get a well-balanced diet of fruits, vegetables, starches and protein than it is to stay perfectly slim.

Why We Love Fat

We're a nation hooked on fat. No wonder—we were raised on cheeseburgers (fat makes up about 50 percent of total calories) and ice cream sundaes (about 60 percent fat). Loving fat may not simply be a result of the American way, though. It may be innate. Adam Drewnowski, Ph.D., director of the University of Michigan's Human Nutrition Program and a leading expert in the psychology of weight loss, believes we have a "fat tooth" that may be more potent than our sweet tooth. He points to U.S. Department of Agriculture surveys that show that the amount of fat in the diet increases during childhood, peaks at adolescence and holds steady throughout adulthood, whereas sugar consumption actually *decreases* with age.

Some people may even be addicted to fat. Dr. Drewnowski's studies of people with eating disorders, as well as obese and depressed people, have convinced him that some of them are addicted to foods containing large amounts of fat and sugar, like chocolate and ice cream. These foods stimulate the brain to produce opioid peptides—substances that create a chemical "high" and a feeling of well-being that these people cannot produce on their own.

Rick Mattes, Ph.D., a nutritionist at the Monell Chemical Senses Center in Philadelphia, suspects that we're born with an instinctive love for fat as well as sweet tastes. "But even if it's innate doesn't mean it can't be modified or controlled," he says. The Japanese, he points out, have preferred a low-fat diet for centuries. He believes that the yearning for fatty foods is often created from a feeling of deprivation. An ice cream sundae suddenly becomes a must when you're on a diet that forbids it!

The Bran Plan staves off those feelings of deprivation by including ice milk and other treats, but we show you how to keep them in check by developing firm control over your diet and food habits. See chapter 8 for tips on overcoming the psychological forces that lead to overeating. Also, your food/schedule diary in the same chapter will give you important clues as to why you overeat.

Yo-yo dieting seems to make people like fattier foods, according to Judith Rodin, Ph.D., chairman of the Psychology Department at Yale University. She gave milk shakes containing varying amounts of fat to a group of yo-yo dieters—women who had lost ten or more pounds at least ten times in their lives—and to a group of women who hadn't yo-yoed. The yo-yo dieters preferred the higher-fat milk shakes and the other group preferred the lower-fat shakes. Her research confirms similar findings in animals.

Outsmarting Fated Fat

After reading that getting fat may be in your genes, that your life-long habits are compounding the problem and that you may even be a fat addict, you can do one of two things: Throw up your hands, declare it hopeless and eat yourself sick or take charge and outsmart fate with some very effective anti-fat weapons.

Weapon number one: A low-fat, high-fiber diet. As we mentioned earlier, you'll lose weight and lower your body fat percentage by simply lowering the fat content of your diet, even without lowering your usual calorie level. The average American eats approximately 40 percent of his or her total calories as fat, whereas 20 percent is the ideal level that really helps you to burn fat and stay healthy. We have designed the Bran Plan for Weight Loss to do the work for you, keeping your diet at no more than 20 percent of calories from fat (about 26 to 36 grams per day). And the Lifelong Bran Plan is also designed to ease you down to about 20 percent of calories from fat (about 30 to 50 grams per day, depending on your total calorie level). So low-fat eating should become second nature to you.

Weapon number two: Exercise. That means walking, jogging, biking, dancing, swimming or almost any other aerobic movement that raises your heart rate for 20 minutes or more. No, we won't accept any of your excuses such as being unable to join a health club or living in the city. You can *always* find a way to exercise, even if it's just an evening stroll. (See chapter 8 for exercise suggestions.) Just be sure to check with your doctor before beginning any new exercise program.

Numerous studies have shown that people who exercise lose more body fat and are more successful at keeping it off. Exercise helps you lose weight in many ways. Most directly, it burns calories, drawing from your fat stores for energy. An hour of moderately paced walking (two miles per hour) can burn anywhere from 165 to more than 300 calories, depending on how much you weigh (the heavier you are, the more calories you burn, because you expend more energy carrying around more weight).

Perhaps even more important for weight loss, exercise increases your muscle mass, which slightly raises your metabolism. That's because your body uses up more calories to maintain muscle than fat, so even while sleeping, you're burning calories at a slightly higher rate. You also lose more calories because exercise seems to reset your "fat thermostat," so that you burn off excess calories more effectively.

Exercise also helps regulate your mood. If you feel better, you'll be less likely to binge. For many people, exercise also regulates appetite, so you eat when you're really hungry—instead of all the time.

Weapon number three: Commitment. If you learn how to eat correctly, stick to it and put yourself back on track after discouraging binges, you will reach the point where eating right becomes automatic, natural and pleasurable. Like most people, you'll have occasional lapses in commitment—but as long as you quickly get back on track, you'll be well rewarded.

Chapter 8 helps you stay committed. Drawing from the experience of our own patients and the experience of leading psychologists specializing in weight loss, we will show you the best methods to help you stick to a healthy, slimming way of eating.

6

The Bran Plan for Weight Loss

O ver the next month, or longer for those who wish to continue, this program can help you lose weight. This won't be the rapid weight loss that many of you may have experienced on previous diets. But the fact that you're trying another diet is testimony enough that *fast weight loss almost guarantees future weight gain.* And you'll like this diet. Although it's low in fat and high in carbohydrates and fiber, you'll still be eating most of the foods you've grown used to, with nothing too strange or difficult to find or to make.

During the first few weeks of the Bran Plan you'll lose weight more quickly, because as your body adjusts to a lower calorie level, it sheds water as well as fat. Then you should settle into a safe and steady weight loss of about ½ to 1 pound per week—which means you will have your best chance ever of really keeping it off.

"But wait a minute," you say, "I want to lose lots of weight immediately." Now before you put down this book, we ask *you* to wait a minute. Take a moment to decide whether you want to lose a few quick pounds that you'll inevitably regain or whether you want to achieve your ideal weight and stay that way while eating like a normal person for the rest of your life. If you make the second choice, read on.

Studies show that people who lose weight slowly and steadily tend to keep it off for years, while those who lose weight quickly regain it in weeks or months. Still, hundreds of diet books persist in promoting quick weight loss, because that's what sells. Usually, they make good on their promise at the expense of their readers, who wind up anemic or tired all the time and unable to tolerate the diet any longer. So the dieters return to their old eating habits, gain all the weight back and continue the pattern with the next new diet book.

The real tragedy of quick weight loss isn't just the virtually guaranteed, demoralizing return of all that fat but the unpleasant truth that *repeated cycles of weight loss and gain (yo-yo dieting) actually make you fatter in the long run.* To lose weight quickly, you have to go on a very low-calorie diet, which sends your body into "starvation mode." In this state, your body desperately clings to every calorie, tucking away more calories as fat and burning as few as it can. In other words, your metabolism (the rate at which we burn calories) slows down. After a few of these diets, your metabolism remains slow even when you're off the diet, making it much easier to gain weight and very much harder to lose it.

Remember: Not only does the Bran Plan for Weight Loss avoid this metabolic slowdown but it also helps veteran dieters raise their sluggish metabolic rates. There's no magic in this, it's simply that we keep calories low enough for you to lose weight but high enough that your body doesn't go into a starvation mode. So your metabolism stays up. For those whose metabolisms have been lowered by previous dieting, this higher calorie level will eventually bring your metabolisms back up.

Healthy, Wealthy and Wise

Added to their effect on metabolism, many diets are also unhealthy and expensive and don't teach you anything about good nutrition. In contrast, the Bran Plan for Weight Loss makes you healthier, isn't expensive and teaches you how to eat right: In effect, it teaches you how food can heal the body rather than destroy it.

You'll start feeling and looking healthier on this plan because it's nutritionally balanced—55 to 65 percent of total calories come from carbohydrates, 15 to 20 percent from fat and 15 to 20 percent from protein. These percentages fall within the guidelines set by the major health organizations. The low fat level—20 percent of total calories (or about 33 grams of fat per day on a 1,500 calorie diet) compared to the nearly 40 percent that the average American consumes—works wonders for you in two ways. Low-fat diets make you lose more body fat while helping protect you from cancer and heart disease.

Numerous studies have shown that given two diets containing exactly the same calorie level, people will lose more body fat on the diet that has a lower percentage of fat. Even more studies show that lowering the percentage of fat in the diet, especially saturated fat (found in coconut and palm oil and animal foods such as butter, red meat and chicken fat), reduces blood cholesterol and the risk of certain cancers.

The Bran Plan for Weight Loss is also chock-full of the cancer-fighting nutrients beta-carotene and vitamin C, and it contains the proper balance of soluble and insoluble fiber to help prevent constipation and other bowel problems, heart disease and certain cancers (see chapter 2 for more on fiber and health).

This plan is as reasonable for your finances as it is good for your health. We give you the option of making your own meals or buying them already prepared. Most homemade items are made up of fairly inexpensive ingredients that you can pick up at the supermarket. The take-out meals will cost a little more because prepared foods are usually more expensive than those you cook yourself.

So that's healthy and wealthy...but this plan will also make you nutrition-wise. It contains a built-in teaching mechanism. While you're losing weight, you are learning to eat the right foods—those low in fat (such as skim milk) and high in fiber (such as vegetables, fruits, whole wheat bread and bran breakfast cereals). To maintain the weight loss, follow the Lifelong Bran Plan outlined in chapter 10.

In contrast to the Bran Plan, after you lose weight on liquid diets or fad diets that revolve around a limited number of foods, you're left wondering what to do next. Since these diets haven't taught you how to eat, it's only human nature to slip and slide back into bad old habits. And as sure as night follows day, back comes the weight.

Variety Is the Spice of Success

The main reason that most diets fail is that they are monotonous and unappealing: three shakes a day or the rigid (and scientifically bogus) rules of combining only certain foods at one time. Can you imagine eating the same foods day after day for the rest of your life? That's what liquid diets and other fad diets demand, setting up even the most resolute dieters for failure. Not having learned good new eating patterns, they go right back to their bad eating habits.

Our motto is *no forbidden foods, only forbidden amounts.* The Bran Plan for Weight Loss contains a wide variety of foods, probably even wider than you're used to. Many of the meals are adventurous and exciting, but never strange or "health food." The only foods we don't include are whole milk dairy foods, high-fat meats and super-rich desserts. That's because we want to keep the fat level low so you'll lose more body fat. Later, in the Lifelong Bran Plan, we'll show you how to slip in a little of these rich foods—occasionally.

The Easiest Eating Plan You'll Ever Follow

Even if an eating plan lives up to all the healthy criteria we mentioned at the beginning of this chapter, it's not going to work if the meals are too difficult to make or the foods too hard to find. So we've tried to make this the easiest eating plan you'll ever follow. Those of you who have the time and inclination to cook—whether that means putting together a salad or sandwich or making a risotto—can turn to the Cook's Plan—28 days of meals you can make yourself (page 64). Very few of them take more than 25 minutes to put together, and many can be made in advance. Those of you who'd rather not cook can follow the Take-Out Plan, where we've developed meals around carry-out, deli and frozen foods (page 93).

Even though we believe this is the most "user friendly" diet ever, addictive or emotional overeating may throw some of you off course. If you find it difficult to stick to the plan, start keeping the food/schedule diary (page 125).

What about Exercise?

Whether it's an after-dinner walk or an advanced aerobics class, exercise will help you to lose weight. But it does more than that; it also works on reshaping your body—replacing the fat with lean muscle tissue. So people who exercise regularly are more successful at keeping weight off permanently.

Exercise influences weight loss in other ways. The more muscle tissue you have, the more calories you burn, even when you aren't exercising and even while you sleep. That's because muscle tissue requires more calories to maintain itself than fat tissue. By building more muscle, you can raise your metabolism. Normally, as we age, we slowly lose muscle, and the body replaces it with fat or flab. Effective exercise can really slow down or prevent this process.

Many people find that exercise also helps by either diminishing appetite or regulating hunger signals so that they feel hungry only when they should be. Exercise also seems to reset your fat thermostat, the threshold that the body uses to decide when to burn off excess calories rather than store them as fat.

Exercise can also put you in a better mood (ever heard of a runner's high?). That's because vigorous exercise triggers the release of endorphins, opiate-like substances in the brain that induce a pleasant sensation of euphoria. You feel better about life in general, better about your body and more in control of your weight. So, people who exercise are able to keep excess weight off better than couch potatoes.

In effect, exercise makes losing weight easier and increases the chances of keeping it off for all the reasons we just mentioned. So we strongly recommend exercise, although it would be wise to consult your physician before you begin.

How to Find Your Weight-Loss Calorie Level

Give two people the same diet for a month or more and one may lose 5 pounds, the other 15 pounds. Differences in metabolism, in the amount of exercise and in the number of times weight has been gained and lost account for the different rates of weight loss among individuals. So there is no magic formula to tell you exactly how many calories you should be consuming to lose a certain amount of weight or how much weight you will lose dieting at a specific calorie level.

Instead, we have given you general guidelines, based on your sex, your previous dieting history and your activity level. Women usually need fewer calories than men partly because they have smaller bodies to feed. If you've been dieting for years, with a history of repeated cycles of weight loss followed by weight gain, your metabolism is probably sluggish. As mentioned earlier, this is because your body goes into "starvation mode." Preparing itself for the next low-calorie bout, it clings to every calorie, storing more calories as fat instead of burning them. And regardless of your calorie level, take a basic multivitamin/mineral tablet for extra insurance on this nutrient-packed plan.

For an at-a-glance summary of what to expect once you've picked your calorie level (and how to adjust that level, if necessary) see the table on page 57.

Who Should Be on a 1,200-Calorie-a-Day Diet?

1. **Women with a long history of dieting.** If you're a woman who has been dieting on and off for years, chances are you have a tough time losing weight even on less than 1,200 calories a day. Cycles of weight loss and gain, even just seven- to ten-pound fluctuations, can lower your metabolism, making it more difficult to lose and easier to gain.

Now it's time to break the cycle. Even if you don't lose much or anything at all for the first few weeks, even if this is more food than you're used to eating, *stick with it.* You'll be rewarded by getting your metabolism back on track, and eventually you'll start shedding the pounds.

2. **Women who are not physically active.** Although exercise is an extremely important accompaniment to dieting, some of you will not be exercising as vigorously as others during these upcoming weeks of the Bran Plan for Weight Loss. Since you won't be burning calories through exercise, you must adhere to the lower-calorie level. However, if the 1,200-calorie plan makes you very hun-

gry, or you find that you are losing more than a pound a week, move up to the 1,500 calorie plan.

Who Should Be on a 1,500-Calorie-a-Day Diet?

1. **Physically active women.** If you exercise almost every day, or have a job where you walk a lot, then you will probably lose weight on 1,500 calories daily. If after two weeks you don't lose, then slip down to the 1,200-calorie level. Do not dip below 1,200 calories. If you're still not losing weight, your metabolism may be slowed down from past dieting and the only way to get your metabolism back on track is by remaining at 1,200 or more calories for a while.

2. **Men who are not physically active.** You may be busy at your office for ten hours a day or more, but if you spend most of that time at a desk, then you're not burning many calories. As you'll discover, exercise is a very important component of any weight-loss plan, but if for some reason you won't be able to exercise enough during the Bran Plan for Weight Loss, then you'll have to stick to 1,500 calories. However, if you are often hungry on this plan, move up to 1,700 calories.

Who Should Be on a 1,700-Calorie-a-Day Diet?

1. **Women who are *very* physically active.** If you exercise for at least one hour daily doing aerobics, jogging or another vigorous sport, or if you are an athlete, you may not need to lose much weight. This daily calorie level should meet your nutrient needs while inducing a pound-a-week weight loss.

2. **Men who are physically active.** If you exercise almost every day, 1,700 calories will meet your nutrient needs while inducing a slow and steady weight loss. If you often feel hungry at this calorie level, you can add a few servings from various food groups (see the note for very physically active men, on page 58).

Note: Some of you may feel that you're eating an awful lot of food, even on the 1,200-calorie plan. The reason you can eat so much is that the diet is low in fat. For instance, you can eat three slices of bread or 1½ cups of pasta and not "use up" any more of your daily calorie quota

Fine-Tuning Your Daily Calorie Level

Expected Weight Loss	Calorie Range		
	1,200	1,500	1,700
Weeks 1 and 2			
1–4 pounds over first 2 weeks	If you're not losing, it's probably because you've been dieting on and off for a while. *Don't* decrease the calorie level. Stick with it and your metabolism will eventually speed up.	If you're not losing, go to 1,200 calories. If you're losing more than 4 pounds and/or you're hungry much of the time, move up to 1,700 calories.	If you're not losing, go to 1,500 calories. If you're losing more than 4 pounds and/or you're hungry much of the time, see "Note for *very* physically active men" on page 58.
Weeks 3 and 4			
½–1½ pounds per week	If you're not losing, stick with it and your metabolism will eventually speed up. If you're losing more than 1½ pounds, go to 1,500 calories.	If you're not losing, scale down to 1,200 calories. If you're losing more than 1½ pounds, go to 1,700 calories.	If you're not losing, scale down to 1,500 calories. If you're losing more than 1½ pounds, see "Note for *very* physically active men" on page 58.
Weeks 5 and 6			
½–1 pound per week	Same as weeks 3 and 4 above.	Same as weeks 3 and 4 above.	Same as weeks 3 and 4 above.

than you once did with a single doughnut.

Note for very physically active men: If you're an athlete or exercise intensely for at least an hour every day, you probably don't have much weight to lose. But if you need to shed some pounds and you feel hungry eating 1,700 calories, add as many servings as you like from the fruit and vegetable group, up to five servings from the breads/grains/cereals group (see the food categories and lists in chapter 10).

Now that you've picked your calorie level for weight loss, turn to the next chapter for the four-week menu plans.

7

28 Days of Weight-Loss Menus

Now that you've decided on your calorie level, you have two 28-day plans to choose from. Make your own meals on the Cook's Plan or eat prepared foods such as frozen microwaveable meals or take-out items from delis and restaurants on the Take-Out Plan.

In either case, here are some important points to keep in mind.

1. Add the Bran Cocktail. Whether you're eating Cook's Plan or Take-Out Plan meals, you must remember to sprinkle on the Bran Cocktail. (Look for the ₢ throughout the meal plans—this Bran Cocktail symbol indicates dishes that are particularly suited to the extra shake of fiber.) Even though both these weight-loss plans are rich in fiber, the Bran Cocktail will ensure that you're meeting the 20-to 35-gram goal. The cocktail will also make the meals more filling, which is always important when you're eating fewer calories than you may be used to.

2. Take a basic multivitamin/mineral tablet while on the Bran Plan for Weight Loss. This is sort of an "insurance plan," to be sure all your basic nutritional needs are met.

3. Stick to the meal plans as closely as possible. In appendix A on page 173, you'll find the recipes for dishes in the Cook's Plan. In appendix B on page 205, you'll find guidelines (including brand names) for suitable types of prepared foods in the Take-Out Plan. *Stick to the recipes and guidelines as closely as possible,* otherwise you may wind up with dishes that are much too high in fat and/or calories.

4. You can switch between the Cook's Plan and the Take-Out Plan. You may want to make some meals and buy others already prepared. If this happens on the same day—for instance, on Day 3 you make breakfast and dinner but want to eat lunch at the diner next to your office building—then make the Cook's Plan breakfast and dinner, and get the Take-Out Plan's lunch. Don't order the Cook's Plan lunch (a tuna salad sandwich at a restaurant or deli counter because it may be much higher in fat and calories than the tuna salad you would prepare yourself using the recipe on page 194.

Or you may switch from one plan to the other for the whole day. For instance, you may follow the entire Cook's Plan on Day 1 and the Take-Out Plan on Days 2 and 3.

5. Keep the day-to-day sequence. When you switch from plan to plan, make sure you are following the days in their correct sequence— no repeating or skipping days. That means you cannot follow Cook's Plan Day 3 on one day, then follow Take-Out Plan Day 3 the next day—you must go to either the Cook's or Take-Out Plan's Day 4. You must stick to the sequence so you don't miss out on vital nutrients. For instance, one day may be a little lower in calcium or beta-carotene, but the next day makes up for it by supplying lots of these nutrients. We have worked it out so that you get an abundance of vital health- and longevity-producing nutrients if you follow the diet in its proper sequence. Also, the total daily calories vary slightly from day to day, but your week's average winds up at 1,200, 1,500 or 1,700 daily. That's another reason to stick to the sequence carefully.

6. Substitution is permitted. Try to stick to the menus as closely as possible. But there are bound to be foods that are hard to find or that you just don't like. So use your common sense and replace them with similar foods (flounder for trout, white rice for brown rice). Most important, stay away from higher-fat substitutions; those extra calories will ruin the weight-loss plan. As a general rule, stay away from foods and meals containing butter, oil, full-fat cheeses, full-fat cream, red meat, or chicken with the skin left on.

If certain fruits are unavailable, out-of-season or simply disliked, you may replace them with fruits of your own choice. Try to replace citrus fruits (such as grapefruit) with other citrus fruits (such as oranges), since we've used these vitamin C–rich fruits to bring you up to recommended levels of vitamin C. The same goes for the beta-carotene–rich orange-fleshed fruits and vegetables, like cantaloupe, mangoes and carrots, and dark green vegetables such as broccoli and spinach.

For variety's sake at breakfast, you can choose among orange juice, orange-pineapple juice and other citrus-based fruit juices. You may substitute any citrus-based juice, as long as one serving contains 100 percent of the RDA (60 milligrams) for vitamin C (ascorbic acid).

7. Buy some berries. This means any of the following alone or mixed: blueberries, raspberries, strawberries or blackberries. Berries are a good source of fiber. If berries are hard to find or out of season, buy them frozen and unsweetened. Keep them in the freezer, taking out only the amount needed. You may add up to a level teaspoon of sugar to berries if they are too tart.

Frozen berries in yogurt make a great brown-bag office snack because the berries keep the yogurt cold for hours.

8. Switch to skim. Every day we've included one or two cups of milk or yogurt to ensure that you get enough bone-building calcium (calcium may also help prevent colon cancer and maintain a normal blood pressure). You may substitute milk for yogurt or vice versa, if you prefer. If you still haven't trained your taste buds for skim milk, substitute ¾ cup 2 percent milk for each cup of skim for the first two weeks. Then switch to 1 percent during the third and fourth weeks. Eventually, whether you continue this weight-loss plan past four weeks or go on the Lifelong Bran Plan, you should make the switch to skim milk. After you get used to skim, you'll never want to drink whole or 2 percent milk again—it will taste oily!

If you're lactose intolerant, you may substitute skim Lactaid milk for milk or yogurt.

9. Be wise about beverages. Aim for at least five glasses of water each day. This is crucial when you are adding the Bran Cocktail (page 31). Besides milk and the morning glass of citrus juice, we haven't included any other beverages. If you're a diet soda drinker, try to have no more than one a day, because these sodas may trigger a desire for sweets. Also, for the same reason, try to limit tea and coffee to once a day, with no more than one teaspoon of sugar. You may drink herbal tea, if you like, but only one cup may be sweetened—the rest must be taken unsweetened. Seltzer water is okay anytime. If you want to have an alcoholic drink, limit it to one glass of wine or one beer or one cocktail no more than three times a week. In exchange for those calories, give up dessert or a slice of bread that day.

10. **You may exchange dinner for lunch.** If it's more convenient, you may have the daily dinner for lunch and the lunch at dinnertime. If, for instance, on Day 7 you are at a business lunch, then it would probably be easier to order the "dinner"—salmon or pasta. Just have the "lunch" of bean salad for dinner.

11. **Eating out is easy.** If your lifestyle demands that you eat out frequently, then try to order foods as similar as possible to those in the Take-Out Plan. Even if nothing on the restaurant's menu closely matches foods on the plan, it's often possible to get the chef to make a few small adjustments so the dish fits into your plan. Remember these basics.

- Always ask for salad dressing on the side, then add the amount listed in the plan.
- Ask for fish, poultry (skin removed) and meat grilled or broiled, not fried, and keep portions to the size of a deck of cards.
- Ask for a baked potato instead of french fries, and a green salad instead of coleslaw.
- Stay away from cheese unless it is fat-free. If the rest of the dish seems to fit the plan (for instance, broccoli with cheese sauce), then order it without cheese.

12. **Sweets are on the menus.** This plan includes sweets several times a week, usually a cookie or frozen yogurt or ice milk. If you like dessert, this should come as a relief. But if you could just as soon do without, then give yourself an extra slice of bread, an extra ½ cup pasta or rice or an extra fruit instead.

If you're prone to bingeing on boxes of cookies or other sweets, then buy just one cookie from a bakery or a single small serving of fresh frozen yogurt instead of a whole box of cookies or a pint of frozen yogurt.

If you love chocolate, you may substitute two Hershey's Kisses for a cookie or ½ cup frozen yogurt or ice milk. Do not buy a large package of Hershey's Kisses—that's inviting trouble. Try to buy just two at a time at a candy counter, or buy the small 1.55-ounce packs, take out two, and put the rest in the back of the freezer. For some people chocolate triggers bingeing. If that's what happens to you, then don't eat it during this weight-loss period. In chapter 8, we'll show you how to bring chocolate back in a controlled way.

13. Vegetarians may substitute. Vegetarians may substitute ½ cup cooked beans, such as chick-peas, black beans and so forth or ¼ cup sliced tofu for each ounce of meat, poultry or fish in the Bran Plan for Weight Loss meals. Tofu is an especially convenient substitute in sandwiches. Tofu is actually higher in fat than turkey breast, one of the common Bran Plan sandwich ingredients, though, so don't add any mayonnaise or any other fat to your tofu sandwich. Tofu slices taste better if you spice them up—sprinkle with a little reduced-sodium soy sauce and spices like ground coriander and pepper, for instance. If you decide to substitute with cooked beans, you also have to eat one less slice of bread, or ⅓ cup less rice or pasta. That's because beans contain both protein (making up for the protein in the substituted meat, poultry or fish dish) and carbohydrate (using up a starch serving).

Note: Within the menu plans that start on the following page, serving sizes are measured either by weight or by volume. Some common measurement conversions follow.

3 teaspoons = 1 tablespoon

2 tablespoons = 1 fluid ounce

8 fluid ounces = 1 cup

2 cups = 1 pint

The Cook's Plan

Week 1

	CALORIES		
	1,200	1,500	1,700

Day 1

Breakfast

	1,200	1,500	1,700
• Bran cereal (p. 213) (Check the box; 1 oz. is usually ½ to 1 cup) with:	1 oz.	1 oz.	1.5 oz.
skim milk	1 cup	1 cup	1 cup
banana	½	½	1
• Orange juice	¾ cup	¾ cup	1 cup

Lunch

	1,200	1,500	1,700
• Turkey sandwich made with:			
turkey breast (p. 227)	2 oz.	3 oz.	3 oz.
mustard	to taste	to taste	to taste
greens (arugula, watercress, etc.)	as desired	as desired	as desired
whole wheat bread (p. 210)	2 slices	2 slices	2 slices
• Apple or pear	1	1	1

Snack

	1,200	1,500	1,700
• Nonfat yogurt (p. 253)	1 cup	1 cup	1 cup
with honey (optional)	1 tsp.	1 tsp.	1 tsp.
• Banana	½	½	1

Dinner

	1,200	1,500	1,700
• Brown rice, cooked (p. 243)	½ cup	½ cup	1 cup
• Bean Burrito (p. 237)	1 recipe	double recipe	double recipe

	1,200	1,500	1,700
with Fresh Tomato Salsa (p. 189)	¼ cup	¼ cup	¼ cup
• Strawberries (fresh or frozen, unsweetened) (p. 234)	1 cup	1 cup	1 cup

Day 2

Breakfast

	1,200	1,500	1,700
• Whole wheat toast (p. 210) with:	1 slice	2 slices	2 slices
peanut butter	½ Tbsp.	1 Tbsp.	1 Tbsp.
banana	½	1	1
honey (optional)	1 tsp.	1 tsp.	1 tsp.
• Skim milk	1 cup	1 cup	1 cup
• Orange juice	¾ cup	¾ cup	1 cup

Lunch

	1,200	1,500	1,700
• Thick Lentil Soup (p. 175)	1 cup	1 cup	2 cups
• Whole wheat bread (p. 210) or	1 slice	2 slices	2 slices
Whole grain nonfat crackers, such as Wasa or Finn Crisps (p. 230)	3	6	6
• Mixed Greens Salad (p. 195)	1 recipe	1 recipe	1 recipe
with Basic Vinaigrette (p. 191)	1 recipe	1 recipe	1 recipe
• Orange	1	1	1

Snack

	1,200	1,500	1,700
• Nonfat yogurt (p. 253) with:	1 cup	1 cup	1 cup
berries or	½ cup	½ cup	½ cup
banana	½	½	½
honey (optional)	1 tsp.	1 tsp.	1 tsp.

(continued)

Week 1—Continued

Day 2—Continued

Dinner

	1,200	1,500	1,700
• Broiled Fish with Garlic-Lemon Marinade (p. 197)	1 recipe (use 3 oz. fish)	1 recipe (use 3 oz. fish)	1 recipe (use 4 oz. fish)
• Broccoli, steamed, with spritz of lemon (p. 201)	1 cup	1 cup	1 cup
• Bran Cocktail Brown Rice 🥫 (p. 181)	½ cup	½ cup	1 recipe
• Strawberry-kiwifruit salad (p. 190) made with:			
strawberries (fresh or frozen, unsweetened) (p. 234)	1 cup	1 cup	1 cup
kiwifruit	1	1	1
Raspberry Topping for Fruit Salad (p. 190)	1 recipe	1 recipe	1 recipe

Day 3

Breakfast

	1,200	1,500	1,700
• Bran Cocktail Muffin 🥫 (p. 182)	1	1	2
• Skim milk	1 cup	1 cup	1 cup
• Berries	½ cup	½ cup	½ cup
• Orange or grapefruit juice	1 cup	1 cup	1 cup

Lunch

	1,200	1,500	1,700
• Tuna sandwich made with: Tuna Salad (p. 194) 🥫 whole wheat bread (p. 210)	1 recipe 2 slices	1 recipe 2 slices	1 recipe 2 slices
• Carrot and celery sticks	4 to 8	4 to 8	4 to 8
• Apple or pear	1	1	1

Dinner

	1,200	1,500	1,700
• Tomato-Bean Stew 🥫 (p. 176)	1½ cups	1½ cups	2 cups

	CALORIES		
	1,200	1,500	1,700
• Brown rice, cooked (p. 243)	½ cup	1 cup	1½ cups
• Mixed Greens Salad (p. 195)	1 recipe	1 recipe	1 recipe
with Honey-Mustard Vinaigrette (p. 191)	1 recipe	1 recipe	1 recipe
• Peach or nectarine	1	1	1

Day 4

Breakfast

	1,200	1,500	1,700
• Bran cereal (p. 213) with:	2 oz.	2 oz.	2 oz.
skim milk	1 cup	1 cup	1 cup
banana	½	1	1
or			
berries	1 cup	1½ cups	1½ cups
• Orange juice	1 cup	1 cup	1 cup

Lunch

	1,200	1,500	1,700
• Peanut butter and jelly sandwich made with:			
peanut butter	1 Tbsp.	1½ Tbsp.	2 Tbsp.
jelly	2 tsp.	2 tsp.	1 Tbsp.
whole wheat bread (p. 210)	2 slices	2 slices	2 slices
• Skim milk	1 cup	1 cup	1 cup
• Carrot and celery sticks	4 to 8	4 to 8	4 to 8
• Nectarine	1	1	1

Dinner

	1,200	1,500	1,700
• Grilled Mustard-Lemon Chicken Breast (p. 178)	1 recipe	1 recipe	1 recipe
• Broccoli, steamed, with spritz of lemon (p. 201)	1 cup	1 cup	1 cup
• Whole wheat roll	1	1	2
with butter or margarine	1 tsp.	1 tsp.	2 tsp.

(continued)

Week 1—Continued

	CALORIES		
	1,200	1,500	1,700

Day 4—Continued

Snack

• Cookie (2-in. diameter)	1	2	2
• Skim milk	1 cup	1 cup	1 cup

Day 5

Breakfast

• Bran Cocktail Muffin (p. 182)	1	1	2
• Skim milk	1 cup	1 cup	1 cup
• Cantaloupe	½	½	½
or			
Mango	1	1	1
• Orange-pineapple juice	½ cup	1 cup	1 cup

Lunch

• Roast beef or ham sandwich made with:			
lean roast beef (p. 207) or ham (p. 226)	3 oz.	3 oz.	3 oz.
lettuce and tomato	as desired	as desired	as desired
mustard	to taste	to taste	to taste
whole wheat bread (p. 210)	2 slices	2 slices	2 slices
• Apple	1	1	1

Dinner

• Spaghetti with tomato sauce made with:			
whole wheat pasta (p. 239)	1½ cups	2 cups	2 cups
Basil-Tomato Sauce (p. 185)	¼ cup	⅓ cup	½ cup
Parmesan cheese	1 Tbsp.	1 Tbsp.	1 Tbsp.
• Mixed Greens Salad (p. 195)	1 recipe	1 recipe	1 recipe
with Basic Vinaigrette (p. 191)	1 recipe	1½ recipes	1½ recipes

	CALORIES		
	1,200	1,500	1,700
• Strawberries (fresh or frozen, unsweetened) (p. 234)	1 cup	1 cup	1 cup
with Yogurt Topping for 🥛 Fruit (p. 204)	1 recipe	1 recipe	1 recipe

Snack

• Graham cracker (preferably whole wheat)	none	1 whole rectangle	2 whole rectangles
with jelly	none	1 tsp.	1 tsp.
• Skim milk	none	none	½ cup

Day 6

Breakfast

• Banana Shake (p. 203) 🥛	1 recipe	1 recipe	1½ recipes

Lunch

• Salmon salad sandwich made with:			
Salmon Salad 🥛 (p. 192)	1 recipe	1 recipe	1 recipe
lettuce and tomato	as desired	as desired	as desired
whole wheat bread (p. 210)	2 slices	2 slices	2 slices
• Cantaloupe	½	½	½
or			
Mango	1	1	1

Dinner

• Oliver's Altogether 🥛 Healthy Stir-Fry (p. 202)	1 recipe	1 recipe (use 3 cups vegetables)	1 recipe (use 3 cups vegetables)
• Brown basmati rice, 🥛 cooked (p. 243)	1 cup	1¼ cups	1½ cups
• Apple or pear	1	1	1

Snack

• Frozen yogurt or ice milk (p. 231)	½ cup	¾ cup	1 cup

(continued)

Week 1—Continued

Day 7

Breakfast

	1,200	1,500	1,700
• Bran cereal (p. 213) with:	1 oz.	1 oz.	1.5 oz.
skim milk	1 cup	1 cup	1 cup
banana	½	½	1
• Orange-pineapple juice	½ cup	1 cup	1 cup

Lunch

	1,200	1,500	1,700
• Three-Bean Salad (p. 177)	1 recipe	1 recipe (use ½ cup chick-peas)	1 recipe (use ¾ cup chick-peas and 1½ tsp. oil)
• Whole wheat pita (p. 212)	1 mini	1 mini	1 regular
• Tomato-Cucumber Salad (p. 195)	1 recipe	1 recipe	1 recipe

Snack

	1,200	1,500	1,700
• Cookie (2-in. diameter)	1	1	1
• Skim milk	½ cup	1 cup	1 cup

Dinner

	1,200	1,500	1,700
• Tropical Glazed Fish (salmon, swordfish or tuna) (p. 197)	1 recipe (use 3 oz. fish)	1 recipe (use 3–4 oz. fish)	1 recipe (use 3–4 oz. fish)
with Black Bean and Dried Fruit Salsa (p. 176)	½ cup	½ cup	½ cup
• Mixed Greens Salad (p. 195)	1 recipe (add a small carrot)	1 recipe (add a small carrot)	1 recipe (add a small carrot)
with Tangerine Vinaigrette (p. 192)	1 recipe	1 recipe	1 recipe

	CALORIES		
	1,200	*1,500*	*1,700*
• Orange-mango or orange-strawberry fruit salad (p. 190) made with:			
orange	1	1	1
mango	1	1	1
or			
strawberries (fresh or frozen, unsweetened) (p. 234)	½ cup	½ cup	½ cup

Week 2

Day 8

Breakfast

• Bran cereal (p. 213)	1 oz.	1.5 oz.	1.5 oz.
with:			
skim milk	1 cup	1 cup	1 cup
berries	1 cup	1 cup	1 cup
or			
banana	½	½	½
• Orange juice	¾ cup	¾ cup	1 cup

Lunch

• Mixed Greens Salad (p. 195)	1 recipe	1 recipe	1 recipe
with Black Bean and Dried Fruit Salsa (p. 176)	¾ cup	¾ cup	1 cup
• Whole wheat bread (p. 210)	1 slice	2 slices	2 slices
or			
Brown rice, cooked (p. 243)	⅓ cup	⅔ cup	⅔ cup
• Kiwi-papaya fruit salad (p. 190) made with:			
kiwifruit	1	1	1
papaya	1	1	1
or			
cantaloupe	⅔	⅔	⅔

(continued)

Week 2—Continued

Day 8—Continued

Dinner

	1,200	1,500	1,700
• Grilled Shrimp with Hot and Sweet Red Peppers (p. 196)	1 recipe (use 6 shrimp)	1 recipe (use 7 shrimp)	1 recipe (use 8 shrimp)
• Tomato Rice (p. 181)	½ recipe	1 recipe	1 recipe (use ⅓ cup plus 2 Tbsp. rice)
• Fruit ice or sorbet (p. 232)	⅓ cup	⅓ cup	¾ cup

Snack

	1,200	1,500	1,700
• Nonfat yogurt (p. 253)	⅓ cup	½ cup	1 cup
• Nectarine or banana	½	½	½

Day 9

Breakfast

	1,200	1,500	1,700
• Bran Cocktail Muffin (p. 182)	1	2	2
• Cantaloupe	½	½	½
or			
Mango	1	1	1
• Orange or grapefruit juice	1 cup	1 cup	1 cup
• Skim milk	1 cup	1 cup	1 cup

Lunch

	1,200	1,500	1,700
• Egg sandwich made with:			
hard-boiled egg	1	1	2
mustard	to taste	to taste	to taste
mayonnaise	1 tsp.	1 tsp.	1 tsp.
lettuce and tomato	as desired	as desired	as desired
whole wheat bread (p. 210)	2 slices	2 slices	2 slices
• Pear	1	1	1

	CALORIES		
	1,200	*1,500*	*1,700*

Dinner
• Pasta with Sun-Dried Tomatoes and Cauliflower (p. 183)	1 recipe	1 recipe	1 recipe (use 1½ cups pasta)
• Mixed green and yellow squash, steamed, with spritz of lemon and sprinkling of salt (p. 201)	1 cup	1 cup	1 cup
• Frozen yogurt or ice milk (p. 231)	none	½ cup	1 cup

Day 10

Breakfast
• Bran cereal (p. 213) with:	1 oz.	1.5 oz.	1.5 oz.
skim milk	1 cup	1 cup	1 cup
banana	½	1	1
• Orange-pineapple juice	½ cup	½ cup	1 cup

Lunch
• Three-Bean Salad (p. 177)	1 recipe	1 recipe (use ¾ cup beans)	1 recipe (use ¾ cup beans)
• Whole wheat pita (p. 212)	1 mini	1 mini	2 mini
• Tomato, sliced	1 med.	1 med.	1 med.
• Apple or pear	1	1	1

Snack
• Nonfat yogurt (p. 253) with:	1 cup	1 cup	1 cup
berries	½ cup	½ cup	½ cup
honey (optional)	1 tsp.	1 tsp.	1 tsp.

(continued)

Week 2–Continued

	CALORIES		
	1,200	**1,500**	**1,700**

Day 10–Continued

Dinner

• Grilled Chicken Strips (p. 178)	1 recipe (use 3 oz. chicken)	1 recipe (use 3 oz. chicken)	1 recipe (use 4 oz. chicken)
over salad greens with:	1 cup	1 cup	1 cup
flour or corn tortilla (p. 234)	1	2	3
A Mano's Tropical Salsa (p. 189)	⅓ cup	⅓ cup	⅓ cup
• Fruit ice or sorbet (p. 232)	½ cup	½ cup	½ cup

Day 11

Breakfast

• Bagel (preferably whole wheat, oat bran or other whole grain) with:	½	1	1
butter or margarine	1 tsp.	2 tsp.	2 tsp.
or			
cream cheese	1 Tbsp.	1½ Tbsp.	1½ Tbsp.
• Cantaloupe	½	½	½
or			
Mango	1	1	1
• Skim milk	1 cup	1 cup	1 cup
• Orange-pineapple juice	¾ cup	¾ cup	1 cup

Lunch

• Thick Lentil Soup (p. 175)	1 cup	1½ cups	2 cups
• Whole wheat bread (p. 210)	1 slice	2 slices	3 slices
or			
Whole grain nonfat crackers, such as Wasa or Finn Crisps (p. 230)	3	6	9
• Apple	1	1	1

| | CALORIES | | |
	1,200	1,500	1,700

Snack
• Nonfat yogurt (p. 253) 🥫	½ cup	1 cup	1 cup
with:			
strawberries	5	5	5
honey (optional)	1 tsp.	1 tsp.	1 tsp.

Dinner
• Broiled fish with Garlic-Lemon Marinade (p. 197)	1 recipe (use 3 oz. fish)	1 recipe (use 3 oz. fish)	1 recipe (use 3–4 oz. fish)
• Yam (sweet potato), baked with Yogurt-Dill Topping (p. 204) 🥫	1 small 2 Tbsp.	1 small 2 Tbsp.	1 med. ⅓ cup
• Carrot-Cabbage Coleslaw (p. 193)	1 recipe	1 recipe	1 recipe
• Strawberry-kiwifruit salad (p. 190) made with:			
strawberries (fresh or frozen, unsweetened) (p. 234)	1 cup	1 cup	1 cup
kiwifruit	1	1	1
Raspberry Topping for Fruit Salad (p. 190)	1 recipe	1 recipe	1 recipe

Day 12

Breakfast
• Bran cereal (p. 213) 🥫	1 oz.	1.5 oz.	1.5 oz.
with:			
skim milk	1 cup	1 cup	1 cup
banana	½	1	1
or			
nectarine	1	2	2
• Orange juice	1 cup	1 cup	1 cup

Lunch
• Turkey sandwich made with:			
turkey breast (p. 227)	2 oz.	3 oz.	3 oz.
mustard	to taste	to taste	to taste

(continued)

Week 2—Continued

	1,200	1,500	1,700
Day 12–Continued			
Lunch–Continued			
greens (arugula, watercress, etc.)	as desired	as desired	as desired
whole wheat bread (p. 210)	2 slices	2 slices	2 slices
• Apricot	3	3	3
or			
Cantaloupe	½	½	½
Dinner			
• Shellfish Risotto (p. 200)	1 recipe	1 recipe (use ⅓ cup rice)	1 recipe (use ⅓ cup rice)
• Mixed Greens Salad (p. 195)	1 recipe	1 recipe	1 recipe
with Basic Vinaigrette (p. 191)	1 recipe	1 recipe	1 recipe
• Orange-grapefruit fruit salad (p. 190) made with:			
orange	1	1	1
grapefruit	½	½	½
Snack			
• Graham cracker (preferably whole wheat)	none	1 whole rectangle	2 whole rectangles
with honey or jam	none	1 tsp.	1 Tbsp.

Day 13

Breakfast			
• Whole wheat toast (p. 210) with:	1 slice	1 slice	1 slice
peanut butter	½ Tbsp.	1 Tbsp.	1 Tbsp.
banana	½	1	1
honey (optional)	1 tsp.	1 tsp.	1 tsp.

	CALORIES		
	1,200	1,500	1,700
• Skim milk	1 cup	1 cup	1 cup
• Orange juice	½ cup	½ cup	½ cup
Lunch			
• Canned minestrone soup (p. 250)	1 cup	1½ cups	1½ cups
• Whole wheat bread (p. 210)	1 slice	2 slices	2 slices
or			
Whole grain nonfat crackers, such as Wasa or Finn Crisps (p. 230)	3	6	6
• Mixed Greens Salad (p. 195)	1 recipe	1 recipe	1 recipe
with Basic Vinaigrette (p. 191)	1 recipe	1 recipe	1 recipe
• Frozen yogurt or ice milk (p. 231)	½ cup	½ cup	½ cup
Snack			
• Bran cereal (p. 213) with:	1 oz.	1 oz.	1 oz.
skim milk	1 cup	1 cup	1 cup
• Nectarine	1	1	1
Dinner			
• Brown rice, cooked (p. 243)	½ cup	½ cup	1 cup
• Bean Burrito (p. 187)	1 recipe	1 recipe (use 2 tortillas)	1 recipe (use ¾ cup beans and 2 tortillas)
with Fresh Tomato Salsa (p. 189)	¼ cup	¼ cup	¼ cup
• Orange-mango fruit salad (p. 190) made with:			
orange	1	1	1
mango	1	1	1

(continued)

——— *CALORIES* ———

	1,200	1,500	1,700

Day 14

Breakfast

	1,200	1,500	1,700
• Bran Cocktail Muffin 🧂 (p. 182)	1	1	2
• Berries	½ cup	1 cup	1 cup
• Grapefruit juice	1 cup	1 cup	1 cup
• Skim milk	1 cup	1 cup	1 cup

Lunch

	1,200	1,500	1,700
• Spinach Salad (p. 194) 🧂	1 recipe	1 recipe (use 2 eggs)	1 recipe (use 2 eggs)
• Whole wheat bread (p. 210)	1 slice	2 slices	2 slices
or			
Whole grain nonfat crackers, such as Wasa or Finn Crisps (p. 230)	3	6	6
• Apple or pear	1	1	1

Dinner

	1,200	1,500	1,700
• Spaghetti with tomato 🧂 sauce made with:			
whole wheat pasta (p. 239)	1½ cups	2 cups	2 cups
Basil-Tomato Sauce (p. 185)	¼ cup	⅓ cup	½ cup
Parmesan cheese	1 Tbsp.	1 Tbsp.	1 Tbsp.
• Broccoli, steamed, with spritz of lemon (p. 201)	1½ cups	1½ cups	1½ cups
or			
Spinach, steamed, with spritz of lemon (p. 201)	¾ cup	¾ cup	¾ cup
• Berries	1 cup	1½ cups	1½ cups

Snack

	1,200	1,500	1,700
• Cookie (2-in. diameter)	1	1	2
• Skim milk	1 cup	1 cup	1 cup

Week 3

	CALORIES		
	1,200	1,500	1,700

Day 15

Breakfast
• Bran cereal (p. 213) with:	1 oz.	1 oz.	1 oz.
skim milk	1 cup	1 cup	1 cup
banana	½	1	1
• Orange-pineapple juice	½ cup	1 cup	1 cup

Lunch
• Mixed Greens Salad (p. 195) with:	1 recipe	1 recipe	1 recipe
chick-peas (canned or cooked from dry)	½ cup	½ cup	¾ cup
Honey-Mustard Vinaigrette (p. 191)	1½ recipes	1½ recipes	1½ recipes
• Whole wheat bread (p. 210)	1 slice	2 slices	2 slices

Dinner
• Oriental Chicken Stir-Fry (p. 179)	1 recipe	1 recipe	1 recipe (use 3½ oz. chicken)
• Brown rice, cooked (p. 243)	½ cup	1 cup	1¼ cups
• Fruit salad (p. 190)	1 cup	1 cup	1 cup

Snack
• Nonfat yogurt (p. 253) with:	½ cup	½ cup	1 cup
banana	½	½	½
honey (optional)	1 tsp.	1 tsp.	1 tsp.

(continued)

Week 3—Continued

	1,200	1,500	1,700
Day 16			
Breakfast			
• Bran cereal (p. 213) with:	1 oz.	1.5 oz.	1.5 oz.
skim milk	1 cup	1 cup	1 cup
peach or nectarine	1	1	1
• Orange-pineapple juice	½ cup	1 cup	1 cup
Lunch			
• Three-Bean Salad (p. 177)	1 recipe	1½ recipes	double recipe
• Whole wheat pita (p. 212)	1 mini	1 mini	1 regular
• Kiwi-orange fruit salad (p. 190) made with:			
kiwifruit	1	1	1
orange	1	1	1
Dinner			
• Pasta with Smoked Salmon and Watercress (p. 199)	1 recipe	1 recipe (use 2½ oz. pasta)	1 recipe (use 2½ oz. pasta)
• Mixed Greens Salad (p. 195)	1 recipe	1 recipe	1 recipe
with vinaigrette (pp. 191–92)	1 recipe	1 recipe	1½ recipes
• Whole wheat bread (p. 210)	none	none	1 slice
• Frozen yogurt or ice milk (p. 231)	½ cup	¾ cup	¾ cup

Day 17

Breakfast

	1,200	1,500	1,700
• Banana Shake (p. 203) 🥤	1 recipe	1 recipe (use 1 banana)	1 recipe (use 1 banana plus 1 cup yogurt, 2 tsp. honey, 8 straw-berries)

Lunch

	1,200	1,500	1,700
• Goat-Cheese Pita Pizza 🥤 (p. 185)	1 recipe	double recipe	double recipe
• Mixed Greens Salad 🥤 (p. 195)	1 recipe	1 recipe	1 recipe
with Basic Vinaigrette (p. 191)	1 recipe	1 recipe	1½ recipes
• Strawberries (fresh or frozen, unsweetened) (p. 234)	1¼ cups	1¼ cups	1¼ cups

Snack

	1,200	1,500	1,700
• Cookie (2-in. diameter)	1	1	1
• Skim milk	1 cup	1 cup	1 cup

Dinner

	1,200	1,500	1,700
• Lentil-Barley Pilaf 🥤 (p. 180)	1½ cups	2 cups	2 cups
with Mint-Yogurt 🥤 Topping (p. 203)	⅓ cup	⅓ cup	½ cup
• Orange	1	1	1

Day 18

Breakfast

	1,200	1,500	1,700
• Bran Cocktail Muffin 🥤 (p. 182)	1	1	2

(continued)

————— *CALORIES* —————

	1,200	1,500	1,700

Day 18—Continued

Breakfast–Continued _____

• Skim milk	1 cup	1 cup	1 cup
• Orange juice	½ cup	1 cup	1 cup
• Apple or pear	1	1	1

Lunch _____

• Peanut butter and jelly sandwich made with:			
peanut butter	1 Tbsp.	1½ Tbsp.	2 Tbsp.
jelly	2 tsp.	2 tsp.	1 Tbsp.
whole wheat bread (p. 210)	2 slices	2 slices	2 slices
• Skim milk	1 cup	1 cup	1 cup
• Carrot and celery sticks	4 to 8	4 to 8	4 to 8
• Apricot	3	3	3
or			
Cantaloupe	½	½	½
• Orange juice	none	none	½ cup
with seltzer water	none	none	to taste

Snack _____

• Cookie (2-in. diameter)	1	2	2
• Skim milk	1 cup	1 cup	1 cup

Dinner _____

• Chicken Fajita (p. 186)	1 recipe	1 recipe (use 2 tortillas)	1 recipe (use 2 tortillas)
with Fresh Tomato Salsa (p. 189)	¼ cup	¼ cup	¼ cup
• Carrot-Cabbage Coleslaw (p.193)	1 recipe	1 recipe	1 recipe

	CALORIES		
	1,200	1,500	1,700
• Kiwifruit	2	2	2
or			
Orange	1	1	1

Day 19

Breakfast
• Bran cereal (p. 213)	1 oz.	1.5 oz.	1.5 oz.
with skim milk	1 cup	1 cup	1 cup
• Cantaloupe	½	½	½
or			
Mango	1	1	1
• Orange-pineapple juice	¾ cup	1 cup	1 cup

Lunch
• Turkey sandwich made with:			
turkey breast (p. 227)	2 oz.	3 oz.	3 oz.
mustard	to taste	to taste	to taste
greens (arugula,	as desired	as desired	as desired
watercress, etc.)			
whole wheat bread (p. 210)	2 slices	2 slices	2 slices
• Apple or pear	1	1	1

Dinner
• All-Bean Chili (p. 188)	1¼ cups	1¼ cups	1¾ cups
• Brown rice, cooked (p. 243)	½ cup	1 cup	1¼ cups
• Mixed Greens Salad (p. 195)	1 recipe	1 recipe	1 recipe
with Basic Vinaigrette (p. 191)	1 recipe	1½ recipes	1½ recipes
• Fruit ice or sorbet (p. 232)	½ cup	½ cup	½ cup

Day 20

Breakfast
• English muffin (preferably whole wheat), toasted (p. 211)	1	1	1

(continued)

Week 3–Continued

	1,200	1,500	1,700

Day 20–Continued

Breakfast–Continued
with:			
peanut butter	1 Tbsp.	1 Tbsp.	1 Tbsp.
banana	½	½	1
honey (optional)	1 tsp.	1 tsp.	1 tsp.
• Skim milk	1 cup	1 cup	1 cup
• Orange juice	¾ cup	1 cup	1 cup

Lunch
• Mixed Greens Salad 🥫 (p. 195)	1 recipe	1 recipe	1 recipe
with:			
chick-peas (canned or cooked from dry)	½ cup	½ cup	¾ cup
Honey-Mustard Vinaigrette (p. 191)	1½ recipes	1½ recipes	1½ recipes
• Whole wheat bread (p. 210)	1 slice	2 slices	2 slices
or			
Whole grain nonfat crackers, such as Wasa or Finn Crisps (p. 230)	3	6	6

Snack
• Nonfat yogurt (p. 253) 🥫	½ cup	1 cup	1 cup
with:			
berries	½ cup	1 cup	1 cup
or			
banana	½	1	1

Dinner
• Tropical Glazed Fish (salmon, swordfish or tuna) (p. 197)	1 recipe (use 3 oz. fish)	1 recipe (use 3–4 oz. fish)	1 recipe (use 3–4 oz. fish)
with A Mano's Tropical Salsa (p. 189)	⅓ cup	⅓ cup	⅓ cup

	CALORIES		
	1,200	1,500	1,700
• Brown basmati rice, ⓤ cooked (p. 243)	½ cup	¾ cup	1 cup
• Strawberry-kiwifruit salad (p. 190) made with:			
strawberries (fresh or frozen, unsweetened) (p. 234)	1 cup	1 cup	1 cup
kiwifruit	1	1	1
Raspberry Topping for Fruit Salad (p. 190)	1 recipe	1 recipe	1 recipe

Day 21

Breakfast

	1,200	1,500	1,700
• Bagel (preferably whole wheat, oat bran or other whole grain) with:	½	1	1
butter or margarine	1 tsp.	2 tsp.	2 tsp.
or			
cream cheese	1 Tbsp.	2 Tbsp.	2 Tbsp.
• Skim milk	1 cup	1 cup	1 cup
• Orange-pineapple juice	¾ cup	1 cup	1 cup
• Peach	1	1	1

Lunch

	1,200	1,500	1,700
• Hamburger (lean ground beef or ground turkey, p. 225), broiled (4 oz. raw, 3 oz. cooked)	1	1	1
or			
Vegetable burger, baked (p. 252) with:	1 patty	1 patty	1 large patty
bun (preferably whole wheat)	1	1	1
ketchup and mustard	to taste	to taste	to taste
• Mixed Greens Salad ⓤ (p. 195)	1 recipe	1 recipe	1 recipe

(continued)

	── CALORIES ──		
	1,200	**1,500**	**1,700**

Day 21—Continued

Lunch—Continued

with vinaigrette (pp. 191–92)	1 recipe	1½ recipes	1½ recipes
• Apple or pear	1	1	1

Dinner

• Yam (sweet potato), baked 🜂 with Yogurt-Dill Topping (p. 204)	1 small 1 recipe	1 med. double recipe	1 large double recipe
• Broccoli, steamed, with spritz of lemon (p. 201)	1½ cups	1½ cups	1½ cups
• Fruit salad (p. 190)	1½ cups	1½ cups	1½ cups

Snack

• Graham cracker (preferably whole wheat)	none	none	1 whole rectangle
with jam	none	none	1 tsp.
• Skim milk	none	none	½ cup

Week 4

Day 22

Breakfast

• Bran cereal (p. 213) 🜂 with:	1 oz.	1.5 oz.	1.5 oz.
skim milk	1 cup	1 cup	1 cup
banana	½	1	1
• Orange juice	¾ cup	¾ cup	¾ cup

Lunch

• Thick Lentil (or Split 🜂 Pea) Soup (p. 175)	1 cup	1½ cups	2 cups
• Whole wheat bread (p. 210)	1 slice	2 slices	2 slices
• Tomato-Cucumber Salad (p. 195)	1 recipe	1 recipe	1½ recipes

	1,200	1,500	1,700
Snack			
• Nonfat yogurt (p. 253) 🥛 with:	1 cup	1 cup	1 cup
berries	1 cup	1 cup	1 cup
honey (optional)	1 tsp.	1 tsp.	1 tsp.
Dinner			
• Agostino's Pasta with Brussels Sprouts (p. 184)	1 recipe	1 recipe	1 recipe (use 1½ cups pasta)
• Any fruit	1	1	1

Day 23

	1,200	1,500	1,700
Breakfast			
• English muffin (preferably whole wheat), toasted (p. 211)	1	1	1
with jam	2 tsp.	2 tsp.	2 tsp.
• Skim milk	1 cup	1 cup	1 cup
• Orange juice	½ cup	1 cup	1 cup
• Cantaloupe	½	½	½
or			
Mango	1	1	1
Lunch			
• Goat-Cheese Pita Pizza 🥛 (p. 185)	1 recipe	1 recipe	1 recipe (use a large pita and ¼ cup plus 1 Tbsp. goat cheese)
• Apple or pear	1	1	1

(continued)

Week 4–Continued

	1,200	1,500	1,700
Day 23–Continued			
Dinner			
• Tomato-Bean Stew (p. 176)	1 cup	1½ cups	2 cups
• Brown rice, cooked (p. 243)	½ cup	1 cup	1 cup
• Mixed Greens Salad (p. 195)	1 recipe	1 recipe	1 recipe
with vinaigrette (pp. 191–92)	1 recipe	1 recipe	1 recipe
• Plum	2	2	2
or			
Peach	1	1	1
Snack			
• Cookie (2-in. diameter)	1	1	2
• Skim milk	none	none	½ cup
Day 24			
Breakfast			
• Poached or boiled egg	1	2	2
• Whole wheat toast (p. 210)	1 slice	2 slices	2 slices
• Orange juice	¾ cup	1 cup	1 cup
• Grapefruit	½	½	½
Lunch			
• Peanut butter and jelly sandwich made with:			
peanut butter	1 Tbsp.	2 Tbsp.	2 Tbsp.
jelly	2 tsp.	1 Tbsp.	1 Tbsp.
whole wheat bread (p. 210)	2 slices	2 slices	2 slices
• Skim milk	1 cup	1 cup	1 cup

	1,200	1,500	1,700
Dinner			
• Oliver's Altogether Healthy Stir-Fry (p. 202)	1 recipe	1 recipe	1 recipe (use 3 cups vegetables)
• Brown basmati rice, cooked (p. 243)	1 cup	1 cup	1½ cups
• Frozen yogurt or ice milk (p. 231)	¾ cup	¾ cup	1 cup
with berries	½ cup	½ cup	½ cup

Day 25

	1,200	1,500	1,700
Breakfast			
• Bran cereal (p. 213) with:	1 oz.	1.5 oz.	1.5 oz.
skim milk	1 cup	1 cup	1 cup
banana	½	1	1
or			
peach	1	1	1
• Orange-pineapple juice	¾ cup	¾ cup	1 cup
Snack			
• Lemon or vanilla nonfat yogurt (p. 253)	½ cup	1 cup	1 cup
Lunch			
• Thick Lentil Soup (p. 175)	1 cup	1½ cups	2 cups
• Whole wheat pita (p. 212)	1 mini	1 regular	1 regular
• Plum	2	2	2
or			
Grapes	15	15	15
Dinner			
• Pasta with Smoked Salmon and Watercress (p. 199)	1 recipe	1 recipe (use 2½ oz. pasta)	1 recipe (use 2½ oz. pasta)

(continued)

Week 4—Continued

	1,200	1,500	1,700

Day 25–Continued

Dinner–Continued

	1,200	1,500	1,700
• Asparagus spears, steamed, with spritz of lemon (p. 201)	7	7	7
• Orange-mango fruit salad (p. 190) made with:			
orange	1	1	1
mango	1	1	1

Day 26

Breakfast

	1,200	1,500	1,700
• Bran Cocktail Muffin (p. 182)	1	1	2
• Skim milk	1 cup	1 cup	1 cup
• Orange juice	¾ cup	1 cup	1 cup
• Nectarine	1	1	1

Lunch

	1,200	1,500	1,700
• Turkey sandwich made with:			
turkey breast (p. 227)	2 oz.	2 oz.	3 oz.
mustard	to taste	to taste	to taste
greens (arugula, watercress, etc.)	3 leaves	3 leaves	3 leaves
whole wheat bread (p. 210)	2 slices	2 slices	2 slices
• Carrot and celery sticks	4 to 8	4 to 8	4 to 8
• Cookie (2-in. diameter)	1	1	2
• Skim milk	1 cup	1 cup	1 cup

Dinner

	1,200	1,500	1,700
• Lentil-Barley Pilaf (p. 180)	1¼ cups	1¾ cups	1¾ cups
with Mint-Yogurt Topping (p. 203)	⅓ cup	½ cup	½ cup
• Tomato-Cucumber Salad (p. 195)	1 recipe	1½ recipes	1½ recipes

	1,200	1,500	1,700
• Cantaloupe-strawberry fruit salad (p. 190) made with:			
cantaloupe	⅓	⅓	⅓
strawberries (fresh or frozen, unsweetened) (p. 234)	½ cup	½ cup	½ cup
Snack			
• Graham cracker (preferably whole wheat)	none	1 whole rectangle	1 whole rectangle
with jam	none	2 tsp.	2 tsp.
• Skim milk	none	½ cup	½ cup

Day 27

Breakfast	1,200	1,500	1,700
• Bran cereal (p. 213) 🧂 with:	1 oz.	1.5 oz.	1.5 oz.
skim milk	1 cup	1 cup	1 cup
banana	1	1	1
• Orange juice	¾ cup	1 cup	1 cup
Lunch			
• Cottage cheese, 1% fat (p. 222)	½ cup	1 cup	1 cup
• Rye crackers (p. 229)	4	4	8
• Fruit salad (p. 190)	1 cup	1 cup	1 cup
Dinner			
• Craig Claiborne's Linguine with Clam Sauce (p. 198)	1 recipe	1 recipe (use 2½ oz. pasta)	1 recipe (use 3 oz. pasta)
• Mixed Greens Salad 🧂 (p. 195)	1 recipe	1 recipe	1 recipe
with vinaigrette (pp. 191–92)	2 tsp.	2 tsp.	1 Tbsp.
• Whole wheat bread (p. 210)	1 slice	2 slices	3 slices
• Frozen yogurt or ice milk (p. 231)	½ cup	½ cup	¾ cup

(continued)

	——— CALORIES ———		
	1,200	**1,500**	**1,700**

Day 27–Continued

Dinner–Continued —

with strawberries (fresh or frozen, unsweetened) (p. 234)	½ cup	¾ cup	1 cup

Day 28

Breakfast ————

• Whole wheat toast (p. 210) with:	2 slices	2 slices	2 slices
butter or margarine	1 tsp.	1 tsp.	1 tsp.
honey or jam	2 tsp.	2 tsp.	1 Tbsp.
• Skim milk	1 cup	1 cup	1 cup
• Orange-pineapple juice	¾ cup	1 cup	1 cup

Snack ————

• Banana Shake (p. 203)	½ recipe	1 recipe	1 recipe (use 1 banana)

Lunch ————

• Thick Lentil (or Split Pea) Soup (p. 175)	1¼ cups	1½ cups	2 cups
• Whole wheat bread (p. 210)	1 slice	2 slices	2 slices
• Papaya or mango	1	1	1

Dinner ————

• Chicken Fajita (p. 186)	1 recipe	1 recipe (use 2 tortillas)	1 recipe (use 2 tortillas)
with Fresh Tomato Salsa (p. 189)	¼ cup	¼ cup	¼ cup
• Carrot-Cabbage Coleslaw (p. 193)	1 recipe	1 recipe	1 recipe
• Frozen yogurt or ice milk (p. 231)	½ cup	½ cup	½ cup

The Take-Out Plan

Week 1

Day 1	1,200	1,500	1,700
Breakfast			
• Bran cereal (p. 213) 🥫 (Check the box; 1 oz. is usually ½ to 1 cup) with:	1 oz.	1 oz.	1.5 oz.
banana	1/2	1/2	1
skim milk	8 oz.	8 oz.	8 oz.
• Orange juice	6 oz.	6 oz.	8 oz.
Lunch			
• Turkey sandwich made with:			
turkey breast (p. 227)	2 oz.	3 oz.	3 oz.
mustard	to taste	to taste	to taste
lettuce and tomato	as desired	as desired	as desired
whole wheat bread (p. 210)	2 slices	2 slices	2 slices
• Apple or pear	1	1	1
Snack			
• Nonfat fruit yogurt 🥫 (p. 253)	8 oz.	8 oz.	8 oz.
Dinner			
• Brown rice, cooked 🥫 (p. 243)	½ cup	1 cup	1¼ cups
• Bean burrito made with: 🥫			
refried beans (p. 235)	½ cup	½ cup	¾ cup
flour or corn tortilla (p. 234)	1	2	2
chopped vegetables	as desired	as desired	as desired
tomato salsa (p. 235)	¼ cup	¼ cup	¼ cup
• Peach	1	1	1

(continued)

——— *CALORIES* ———

	1,200	1,500	1,700

Day 2

Breakfast

• Whole wheat toast (p. 210) with:	1 slice	2 slices	2 slices
banana	½	1	1
honey or jam	1 tsp.	1 tsp.	1 tsp.
peanut butter	½ Tbsp.	1 Tbsp.	1 Tbsp.
or			
butter or margarine	1 tsp.	2 tsp.	2 tsp.
• Skim milk	8 oz.	8 oz.	8 oz.
• Orange juice	6 oz.	6 oz.	8 oz.
• Nectarine	1	1	1

Lunch

• Lentil or bean soup (p. 250)	1 cup	1 cup	2 cups
• Whole wheat bread (p. 210)	1 slice	2 slices	2 slices
• Green salad	1 cup or more	1 cup or more	1 cup or more
with:			
regular salad dressing (p. 247)	1 tsp.	2 tsp.	2 tsp.
or			
reduced-calorie salad dressing (p. 245)	1 Tbsp.	1 Tbsp.	1 Tbsp.
• Orange	1	1	1

Snack

• Nonfat fruit yogurt (p. 253)	8 oz.	8 oz.	8 oz.

Dinner

• Broiled fish	3 oz.	3 oz.	4 oz.
• Broccoli, steamed, with spritz of lemon (p. 201)	1 cup	1 cup	1 cup

	CALORIES		
	1,200	**1,500**	**1,700**
• Brown rice, cooked 🥫 (p. 243)	½ cup	½ cup	1 cup
• Fruit salad	1 cup	1 cup	1 cup

Day 3

Breakfast

• Bran muffin (p. 238) (avoid "jumbo" muffins)	1 small	2 small or 1 med.	2 small or 1 med.
• Nonfat fruit yogurt 🥫 (p. 253)	8 oz.	8 oz.	8 oz.
• Orange or grapefruit juice	8 oz.	8 oz.	8 oz.

Lunch

• Salad bar tuna salad made 🥫 with:			
tuna, plain	¼ cup	¼ cup	¼ cup
Romaine lettuce or spinach	1 cup or more	1 cup or more	1 cup or more
carrot sticks	4 to 8	4 to 8	4 to 8
regular salad dressing (p. 247)	2 tsp.	1 Tbsp.	1 Tbsp.
or			
reduced-calorie salad dressing (p. 245)	1 Tbsp.	1 to 2 Tbsp.	1 to 2 Tbsp.
• Whole wheat bread (p. 210)	2 slices	2 slices	2 slices
• Cantaloupe	½	½	½

Dinner

• Vegetarian chili (p. 236) 🥫 or baked beans (p. 206)	1 cup	1½ cups	1½ cups
• Brown rice, cooked 🥫 (p. 243)	½ cup	1 cup	1¼ cups
• Green salad 🥫	1 cup or more	1 cup or more	1 cup or more

(continued)

Week 1–Continued

Day 3–Continued

Dinner–Continued

	1,200	1,500	1,700
with:			
regular salad dressing (p. 247)	1 tsp.	2 tsp.	2 tsp.
or			
reduced-calorie salad dressing (p. 245)	1 Tbsp.	1 to 2 Tbsp.	1 to 2 Tbsp.
• Peach or nectarine	1	1	1

Day 4

Breakfast

	1,200	1,500	1,700
• Bran cereal (p. 213)	2 oz.	2 oz.	2 oz.
with:			
skim milk	8 oz.	8 oz.	8 oz.
banana	½	1	1
or			
berries (p. 234)	1 cup	1 cup	1 cup
• Orange juice	8 oz.	8 oz.	8 oz.

Lunch

	1,200	1,500	1,700
• Peanut butter and jelly sandwich made with:			
peanut butter	1 Tbsp.	1½ Tbsp.	2 Tbsp.
jelly	2 tsp.	2 tsp.	1 Tbsp.
whole wheat bread (p. 210)	2 slices	2 slices	2 slices
• Skim milk	8 oz.	8 oz.	8 oz.
• Carrot and celery sticks	4 to 8	4 to 8	4 to 8
• Nectarine or apple	1	1	1

	1,200	1,500	1,700
Dinner			
• Frozen chicken and vegetable entrée (p. 223)	1 (240–60 calories, 5 grams fat or less)	1 (300–330 calories, 7 grams fat or less)	1 (300–330 calories, 7 grams fat or less)
• Whole wheat roll with butter or margarine	1 1 tsp.	1 1 tsp.	2 2 tsp.
Snack			
• Cookie (2-in. diameter)	1	2	2
• Skim milk	8 oz.	8 oz.	8 oz.
• Any fruit	none	none	1

Day 5

	1,200	1,500	1,700
Breakfast			
• Bran muffin (p. 238) (avoid "jumbo" muffins)	1 small	1 small	2 small or 1 med.
• Skim milk	8 oz.	8 oz.	8 oz.
• Cantaloupe	½	½	½
• Orange-pineapple juice	4 oz.	8 oz.	8 oz.
Lunch			
• Roast beef or ham sandwich made with:			
lean roast beef (p. 207) or ham (p. 226)	3 oz.	3 oz.	3 oz.
mustard	to taste	to taste	to taste
lettuce and tomato	as desired	as desired	as desired
whole wheat bread (p. 210)	2 slices	2 slices	2 slices
• Apple	1	1	1

(continued)

Week 1–Continued

Day 5–Continued

Dinner

	1,200	1,500	1,700
• Spaghetti with tomato sauce made with:			
spaghetti (preferably whole wheat) (p. 239)	1 cup	2 cups	2 cups
tomato sauce (p. 240)	⅓ cup	½ cup	½ cup
Parmesan cheese	1 tsp.	1 Tbsp.	1 Tbsp.
• Green salad with:	1½ cups	1½ cups	1½ cups
regular salad dressing (p. 247)	2 tsp.	1 Tbsp.	1 Tbsp.
or			
reduced-calorie salad dressing (p. 245)	1 Tbsp.	1 to 2 Tbsp.	1 to 2 Tbsp.
• Strawberries (fresh or frozen, unsweetened) (p. 234)	1 cup	1 cup	1 cup
with vanilla nonfat yogurt (p. 253)	4 oz.	4 oz.	4 oz.

Snack

	1,200	1,500	1,700
• Graham cracker (preferably whole wheat)	none	1 whole rectangle	2 whole rectangles
with jelly	none	1 tsp.	2 tsp.
• Skim milk	none	none	4 oz.

Day 6

Breakfast

	1,200	1,500	1,700
• Vanilla nonfat yogurt (p. 253)	8 oz.	8 oz.	8 oz.
with banana	½	½	½

	1,200	1,500	1,700

Lunch _____

- Salad bar salad made 🧂
  with:

tuna, plain	¼ cup	¼ cup	¼ cup
Romaine lettuce or spinach	1 cup	1 cup	1 cup
carrot sticks	4 to 8	4 to 8	4 to 8
regular salad dressing (p. 247)	2 tsp.	1 Tbsp.	1 Tbsp.
or			
reduced-calorie salad dressing (p. 245)	1 Tbsp.	1 to 2 Tbsp.	1 to 2 Tbsp.

- Whole wheat bread (p. 210) — 2 slices / 2 slices / 2 slices
- Cantaloupe — ½ / ½ / ½
- Orange juice — 6 oz. / 6 oz. / 6 oz.
  with seltzer water — to taste / to taste / to taste

Dinner _____

- Stir-fried vegetables 🧂
  and rice made with:

frozen vegetable entrée (p. 252)	1	1	1
brown rice, cooked (p. 243)	1 cup	1 cup	1 cup

- Apple or pear — 1 / 1 / 1

Snack _____

- Frozen yogurt or ice milk (p. 231) — ½ cup / ¾ cup / 1 cup

Day 7

Breakfast _____

- Bran cereal (p. 213) 🧂 — 1 oz. / 1 oz. / 1.5 oz.
  with:

skim milk	8 oz.	8 oz.	8 oz.
banana	½	½	½

- Orange-pineapple juice — 4 oz. / 8 oz. / 8 oz.

(continued)

Week 1—Continued

	1,200	1,500	1,700

Day 7—Continued

Lunch

	1,200	1,500	1,700
• Three-bean salad made 🥫 with chick-peas, kidney beans and green beans, or other combinations (p. 206)	1¼ cups	1½ cups	1¾ cups
or Lentil or bean soup 🥫 (p. 250)	1 cup	1¼ cups	1½ cups
• Whole wheat pita (p. 212)	1 mini	1 mini	1 regular
or Whole wheat bread (p. 210)	1 slice	1 slice	2 slices
• Tomato-cucumber salad	1 cup	1 cup	1 cup
or Green salad 🥫 with:	1 cup	1 cup	1 cup
regular salad dressing (p. 247)	2 tsp.	2 tsp.	2 tsp.
or reduced-calorie salad dressing (p. 245)	1 Tbsp.	1 Tbsp.	1 Tbsp.

Snack

	1,200	1,500	1,700
• Cookie (2-in. diameter)	1	1	1
• Skim milk	4 oz.	8 oz.	8 oz.

Dinner

	1,200	1,500	1,700
• Grilled fish (salmon, tuna or swordfish)	3 oz.	3–4 oz.	3–4 oz.
• Potato, baked	1 small	1 med.	1 med.
with sour cream (preferably reduced-fat)	½ Tbsp.	1 Tbsp.	1 Tbsp.
• Broccoli, steamed, with spritz of lemon (p. 201)	½ cup	½ cup	½ cup
• Fruit salad	1¼ cups	1¼ cups	1¼ cups

Week 2

Day 8

Breakfast	1,200	1,500	1,700
• Bran cereal (p. 213)	1 oz.	1.5 oz.	1.5 oz.
• Skim milk	8 oz.	8 oz.	8 oz.
• Berries	1 cup	1 cup	1 cup
or			
Banana	½	½	½
• Orange juice	6 oz.	6 oz.	8 oz.

Lunch			
• Vegetarian beans (p. 206)	¾ cup	¾ cup	1 cup
• Whole wheat bread (p. 210)	1 slice	2 slices	2 slices
or			
Brown rice, cooked (p. 243)	⅓ cup	⅔ cup	⅔ cup
• Fruit salad	1 cup	1 cup	1 cup

Dinner			
• Shrimp and vegetable frozen entrée (200–230 calories) (p. 249)	1	1	1
with brown rice, cooked (p. 243)	1 cup	1 cup	1½ cups
• Fruit ice or sorbet (p. 232)	⅓ cup	⅓ cup	¾ cup

Snack			
• Vanilla nonfat yogurt (p. 253)	4 oz.	4 oz.	8 oz.
• Nectarine	1	1	1
or			
Banana	½	½	½

(continued)

Week 2—Continued

	1,200	1,500	1,700

Day 9

Breakfast

• Bran muffin (p. 238) (avoid "jumbo" muffins)	1 small	2 small or 1 med.	2 small or 1 med.
• Cantaloupe	½	½	½
or			
Mango	1	1	1
• Orange or grapefruit juice	8 oz.	8 oz.	8 oz.
• Skim milk	8 oz.	8 oz.	8 oz.

Lunch

• Egg sandwich made with:			
hard-boiled egg, sliced	1	1	2
or			
chopped eggs from salad bar	¼ cup	¼ cup	½ cup
mustard	to taste	to taste	to taste
mayonnaise	1 tsp.	1 tsp.	1 tsp.
lettuce and tomato	as desired	as desired	as desired
whole wheat bread (p. 210)	2 slices	2 slices	2 slices
• Apple or pear	1	1	1

Dinner

• Pasta with tomato sauce made with:			
pasta (preferably whole wheat) (p. 239)	2 cups	2 cups	2½ cups
tomato sauce (p. 240)	⅓ cup	½ cup	½ cup
Parmesan cheese	1½ Tbsp.	1½ Tbsp.	1½ Tbsp.
• Vegetables, steamed, with spritz of lemon (p. 201)	½ cup	1 cup	1 cup
• Fruit	1	1	1
• Frozen yogurt or ice milk (p. 231)	none	½ cup	1 cup

	1,200	1,500	1,700

Day 10

Breakfast

	1,200	1,500	1,700
• Bran cereal (p. 213) with:	1 oz.	1.5 oz.	1.5 oz.
skim milk	8 oz.	8 oz.	8 oz.
banana	1	1	1
• Orange-pineapple juice	4 oz.	6 oz.	8 oz.

Lunch

	1,200	1,500	1,700
• Three-bean salad made with chick-peas, kidney beans and green beans, or other combinations (p. 206)	1¼ cups	1½ cups	1¾ cup
• Whole wheat pita (p. 212)	1 mini	1 mini	2 mini
• Tomato slices	3 to 6	3 to 6	3 to 6
• Apple or pear	1	1	1

Snack

	1,200	1,500	1,700
• Nonfat fruit yogurt (p. 253)	8 oz.	8 oz.	8 oz.

Dinner

	1,200	1,500	1,700
• Chicken fajita (p. 238)	1	1 (plus 1 tortilla)	1 (plus 2 tortillas)
with tomato salsa (p. 235)	¼ cup	½ cup	½ cup
• Green salad	1 cup or more	1 cup or more	1 cup or more
with: regular salad dressing (p. 247)	2 tsp.	2 tsp.	2 tsp.
or reduced-calorie salad dressing (p. 245)	1 Tbsp.	1 Tbsp.	1 Tbsp.
• Fruit ice or sorbet (p. 232)	½ cup	½ cup	½ cup

(continued)

	──── CALORIES ────		
	1,200	1,500	1,700

Day 11

Breakfast

	1,200	1,500	1,700
• Bagel (preferably whole wheat, oat bran or other whole grain) with:	½	1	1
butter or margarine	1 tsp.	2 tsp.	2 tsp.
or			
cream cheese	1 Tbsp.	1½ Tbsp.	1½ Tbsp.
• Mango	1	1	1
or			
Cantaloupe	½	½	½
• Skim milk	8 oz.	8 oz.	8 oz.
• Orange juice	6 oz.	6 oz.	8 oz.

Lunch

	1,200	1,500	1,700
• Lentil soup (p. 250)	1 cup	1½ cups	2 cups
• Whole wheat bread (p. 210)	1 slice	2 slices	3 slices
• Apple	1	1	1

Snack

	1,200	1,500	1,700
• Nonfat fruit yogurt (p. 253)	4 oz.	8 oz.	8 oz.

Dinner

	1,200	1,500	1,700
• Broiled, baked, steamed or grilled fish	3 oz.	3 oz.	3–4 oz.
• Vegetables, steamed, with spritz of lemon (p. 201)	1 cup	1 cup	1 cup
• Yam (sweet potato) or potato, baked	1 med.	1 med.	1 med.
with sour cream (preferably reduced-fat)	1 Tbsp.	1 Tbsp.	1 Tbsp.
• Green salad	1 cup or more	1 cup or more	1 cup or more

	1,200	1,500	1,700
with: regular salad dressing (p. 247)	2 tsp.	2 tsp.	2 tsp.
or			
reduced-calorie salad dressing (p. 245)	1 Tbsp.	1 Tbsp.	1 Tbsp.
• Fruit salad	1¼ cups	1¼ cups	1¼ cups

Day 12

Breakfast

	1,200	1,500	1,700
• Bran cereal (p. 213) with:	1 oz.	1.5 oz.	1.5 oz.
skim milk	8 oz.	8 oz.	8 oz.
banana	½	1	1
• Orange juice	8 oz.	8 oz.	8 oz.

Lunch

	1,200	1,500	1,700
• Turkey sandwich made with: turkey breast (p. 227) mustard lettuce and tomato whole wheat bread (p. 210)	2 oz. to taste as desired 2 slices	3 oz. to taste as desired 2 slices	3 oz. to taste as desired 2 slices
• Apricot	3	3	3
or			
Cantaloupe	½	½	½

Dinner

	1,200	1,500	1,700
• Shrimp and vegetable stir-fry frozen entrée, including rice	1 serving (350 calories or less, 6 grams fat or less)	1 serving (450 calories or less, 6 grams fat or less)	1 serving (450 calories or less, 6 grams fat or less)
or			
Frozen shrimp and vegetable stir-fry entrée, not including rice (200 calories or less, 5 grams fat or less) (p. 249)	1	1	1

(continued)

	———— CALORIES ————		
	1,200	**1,500**	**1,700**

Day 12—Continued

Dinner—Continued

plus:			
brown rice, cooked (p. 243)	½ cup	1 cup	1½ cups
vegetables, steamed, with spritz of lemon (p. 201) or tamari sauce	1 cup or more	1 cup or more	1 cup or more
• Fruit salad	1 cup	1 cup	1 cup

Snack

• Graham cracker (preferably whole wheat)	1 whole rectangle	2 whole rectangles	3 whole rectangles
with honey or jam	none	1 tsp.	1 Tbsp.
• Skim milk	8 oz.	8 oz.	8 oz.

Day 13

Breakfast

• Whole wheat toast (p. 210) with:	1 slice	1 slice	1 slice
banana	½	1	1
honey or jam	1 tsp.	1 tsp.	1 tsp.
peanut butter	½ Tbsp.	1 Tbsp.	1 Tbsp.
or			
butter or margarine	1 tsp.	1 tsp.	1 tsp.
• Skim milk	8 oz.	8 oz.	8 oz.
• Orange juice	4 oz.	4 oz.	4 oz.

Lunch

• Minestrone soup (p. 250)	1 cup	1½ cups	1½ cups
• Whole wheat bread (p. 210)	1 slice	2 slices	2 slices
• Green salad	1 cup or more	1 cup or more	1 cup or more
with:			
regular salad dressing (p. 247)	1 tsp.	2 tsp.	2 tsp.

	CALORIES		
	1,200	1,500	1,700

	1,200	1,500	1,700
or reduced-calorie salad dressing (p. 245)	1 Tbsp.	1 to 2 Tbsp.	1 to 2 Tbsp.
• Frozen yogurt or ice milk (p. 231)	½ cup	½ cup	½ cup

Snack

	1,200	1,500	1,700
• Nonfat fruit yogurt (p. 253)	8 oz.	8 oz.	8 oz.
• Banana	1	1	1

Dinner

	1,200	1,500	1,700
• Bean burrito made with: refried beans (p. 235)	½ cup	½ cup	¾ cup
flour or corn tortilla (p. 234)	1	2	2
chopped vegetables	as desired	as desired	as desired
tomato salsa (p. 235)	¼ cup	¼ cup	¼ cup
• Brown rice, cooked (p. 243)	½ cup	½ cup	1 cup
• Fruit salad	1½ cups	1½ cups	1½ cups

Day 14

Breakfast

	1,200	1,500	1,700
• Bran muffin (p. 238) (avoid "jumbo" muffins)	1 small	1 small	2 small or 1 med.
• Peach	1	1	1
• Grapefruit juice	8 oz.	8 oz.	8 oz.
• Skim milk	8 oz.	8 oz.	8 oz.

Lunch

	1,200	1,500	1,700
• Spinach salad made with: spinach	1 cup	1 cup	1 cup
egg	1	2	2

(continued)

——— CALORIES ———

	1,200	1,500	1,700

Day 14–Continued

Lunch–Continued

	1,200	1,500	1,700
regular salad dressing (p. 247)	2 tsp.	1 Tbsp.	1 Tbsp.
or			
reduced-calorie salad dressing (p. 245)	1 Tbsp.	1 to 2 Tbsp.	1 to 2 Tbsp.
• Whole wheat bread (p. 210)	1 slice	2 slices	2 slices
or			
Whole grain nonfat crackers, such as Wasa or Finn Crisps (p. 230)	3	6	6
• Mango	1	1	1
or			
Cantaloupe	½	½	½

Dinner

	1,200	1,500	1,700
• Pasta with tomato sauce made with:			
pasta (preferably whole wheat) (p. 239)	1½ cups	2 cups	2 cups
meatless tomato sauce (p. 240)	¼ cup	⅓ cup	½ cup
Parmesan cheese	1 Tbsp.	1 Tbsp.	1 Tbsp.
• Broccoli, steamed, with spritz of lemon (p. 201)	1½ cups	1½ cups	1½ cups
or			
Spinach, steamed, with spritz of lemon (p. 201)	¾ cup	¾ cup	¾ cup
• Any fruit	1	1	1

Snack

	1,200	1,500	1,700
• Cookie (2-in. diameter)	1	1	2
• Skim milk	8 oz.	8 oz.	8 oz.

Week 3

CALORIES

	1,200	1,500	1,700

Day 15

Breakfast

	1,200	1,500	1,700
• Bran cereal (p. 213) with:	1 oz.	1 oz.	1 oz.
skim milk	8 oz.	8 oz.	8 oz.
banana	½	1	1
• Orange juice	4 oz.	8 oz.	8 oz.

Lunch

	1,200	1,500	1,700
• Green salad with:	1½ cups	1½ cups	1½ cups
chick-peas, canned	½ cup	½ cup	¾ cup
regular salad dressing (p. 247)	2 tsp.	2 tsp.	1 Tbsp.
or			
reduced-calorie salad dressing (p. 245)	1 Tbsp.	1 to 2 Tbsp.	1 to 2 Tbsp.
• Whole wheat bread (p. 210)	1 slices	2 slices	2 slices

Dinner

	1,200	1,500	1,700
• Chicken-vegetable entrée using:			
Chinese take-out (request very little oil)	1 pint, including 3 oz. chicken	1 pint, including 3 oz. chicken	1 pint, including 3 oz. chicken
or			
chicken-vegetable frozen entrée (p. 223)	1 (250–80 calories, 9 grams fat or less)	1 (250–80 calories, 9 grams fat or less)	1 (300–340 calories, 9 grams fat or less)
plus brown rice, cooked (p. 243)	½ cup	1 cup	1¼ cups
• Fruit salad	1 cup	1 cup	1 cup

(continued)

Week 3—Continued

	1,200	1,500	1,700
Day 15—Continued			
Snack			
• Vanilla nonfat yogurt (p. 253)	4 oz.	4 oz.	8 oz.
• Nectarine or other fruit	1	1	1
Day 16			
Breakfast			
• Bran cereal (p. 213) with:	1 oz.	1.5 oz	1.5 oz.
skim milk	8 oz.	8 oz.	8 oz.
banana	1	1	1
• Orange juice	4 oz.	8 oz.	8 oz.
Lunch			
• Three-bean salad made with chick-peas, kidney beans and green beans, or other combinations (p. 206)	1¼ cups	1½ cups	1¾ cups
or			
Lentil or bean soup (p. 250)	1 cup	1½ cups	2 cups
• Whole wheat pita (p. 212)	1 mini	2 mini	2 regular
or			
Whole wheat bread (p. 210)	1 slice	2 slices	3 slices
• Fruit salad	1 cup	1 cup	1 cup
Dinner			
• Pasta with seafood frozen entrée (250–70 calories) (p. 249)	1	1	1
• Green salad with:	1 cup	1 cup	1 cup
regular salad dressing (p. 247)	2 tsp.	2 tsp.	1 Tbsp.
or			
reduced-calorie salad dressing (p. 245)	1 Tbsp.	1 to 2 Tbsp.	1 to 2 Tbsp.

	CALORIES		
	---	---	---
	1,200	1,500	1,700
• Frozen yogurt or ice milk (p. 231)	½ cup	¾ cup	1 cup

Day 17

Breakfast
• Vanilla nonfat yogurt (p. 253)	8 oz.	8 oz.	8 oz.
• Banana	½	1	1
• Orange juice	8 oz.	8 oz.	8 oz.

Lunch
• Vegetarian pizza	1 slice	1 slice	2 slices
• Green salad with:	1 cup	1 cup	1 cup
regular salad dressing (p. 247)	2 tsp.	2 tsp.	1 Tbsp.
or			
reduced-calorie salad dressing (p. 245)	1 Tbsp.	1 to 2 Tbsp.	1 to 2 Tbsp.
• Strawberries (fresh or frozen, unsweetened) (p. 234)	1 cup	1 cup	1 cup
with vanilla nonfat yogurt (p. 253)	2 oz.	2 oz.	2 oz.

Snack
• Cookie (2-in. diameter)	1	1	2
• Skim milk	8 oz.	8 oz.	8 oz.

Dinner
• Lentil-rice pilaf from mix (p. 245)	1½ cups	2 cups	2 cups
or			
Lentil soup (p. 250)	1 cup	1½ cups	1½ cups
plus brown rice, cooked (p. 243)	1 cup	1½ cups	1¼ cups
• Orange	1	1	1

(continued)

——— *CALORIES* ———

	1,200	1,500	1,700

Day 18

Breakfast

	1,200	1,500	1,700
• Bran muffin (p. 238) (avoid "jumbo" muffins)	1 small	1 small	2 small or 1 med.
• Skim milk	8 oz.	8 oz.	8 oz.
• Orange juice	4 oz.	8 oz.	8 oz.
• Peach	1	1	1

Lunch

	1,200	1,500	1,700
• Peanut butter and jelly sandwich made with:			
peanut butter	1 Tbsp.	1½ Tbsp.	2 Tbsp.
jelly	2 tsp.	2 tsp.	1 Tbsp.
whole wheat bread (p. 210)	2 slices	2 slices	2 slices
• Skim milk	8 oz.	8 oz.	8 oz.
• Carrot and celery sticks	4 to 8	4 to 8	4 to 8
• Apple	1	1	1

Snack

	1,200	1,500	1,700
• Cookie (2-in. diameter)	1	2	2
• Skim milk	8 oz.	8 oz.	8 oz.

Dinner

	1,200	1,500	1,700
• Chicken fajita (p. 238)	1	1	1
with tomato salsa (p. 235)	¼ cup	½ cup	½ cup
• Green salad with:	2 cups	2 cups	2 cups
regular salad dressing (p. 247)	2 tsp.	2 tsp.	1 Tbsp.
or			
reduced-calorie salad dressing (p. 245)	1 Tbsp.	1 to 2 Tbsp.	1 to 2 Tbsp.
• Orange	1	1	1

	1,200	1,500	1,700

Day 19

Breakfast

• Bran cereal (p. 213)	1 oz.	1.5 oz.	2 oz.
with skim milk	8 oz.	8 oz.	8 oz.
• Cantaloupe	½	½	½
• Grapefruit juice	6 oz.	8 oz.	8 oz.

Lunch

• Turkey sandwich made with:			
turkey breast (p. 227)	2 oz.	3 oz.	3 oz.
mustard	to taste	to taste	to taste
mayonnaise	1 tsp.	1 tsp.	1 tsp.
lettuce and tomato	as desired	as desired	as desired
whole wheat bread (p. 210)	2 slices	2 slices	2 slices
• Apple or pear	1	1	1

Dinner

• Vegetarian chili (p. 236)	1 cup	1 cup	1½ cups
• Brown rice, cooked (p. 243)	½ cup	1 cup	1¼ cups
• Green salad with:	1½ cups	1½ cups	1½ cups
regular salad dressing (p. 247)	2 tsp.	2 tsp.	1 Tbsp.
or			
reduced-calorie salad dressing (p. 245)	1 Tbsp.	1 Tbsp.	1 Tbsp.
• Fruit ice or sorbet (p. 232)	½ cup	½ cup	½ cup

Day 20

Breakfast

• English muffin (preferably whole wheat), toasted (p. 211)	1	1	1

(continued)

Week 3—Continued

	CALORIES		
	1,200	1,500	1,700

Day 20—Continued

Breakfast–Continued

with:			
banana	½	½	½
honey or jam	1 tsp.	1 tsp.	1 tsp.
peanut butter	1 Tbsp.	1 Tbsp.	1 Tbsp.
or			
butter or margarine	1 tsp.	1 tsp.	1 tsp.
• Cantaloupe	½	½	½
• Skim milk	8 oz.	8 oz.	8 oz.
• Orange juice	6 oz.	8 oz.	8 oz.

Lunch

• Salad bar salad made with:			
spinach and lettuce	1½ cups	1½ cups	1½ cups
carrots, green peppers or other fresh vegetables	1 cup	1 cup	1 cup
chick-peas	½ cup	½ cup	¾ cup
with:			
regular salad dressing (p. 247)	1 Tbsp.	1 Tbsp.	1 Tbsp.
or			
reduced-calorie salad dressing (p. 245)	1 to 2 Tbsp.	1 to 2 Tbsp.	1 to 2 Tbsp.
• Whole wheat bread (p. 210)	1 slice	2 slices	2 slices
or			
Whole grain nonfat crackers, such as Wasa or Finn Crisps (p. 230)	3	6	6

Snack

• Nonfat fruit yogurt (p. 253)	4 oz.	8 oz.	8 oz.

Dinner

• Grilled or broiled fish	3 oz.	3–4 oz.	3–4 oz.
with chutney	1 Tbsp.	1 Tbsp.	1 Tbsp.

	CALORIES		
	1,200	*1,500*	*1,700*
• Brown rice, cooked 🔲 (p. 243)	½ cup	¾ cup	1 cup
• Fruit salad	1 cup	1 cup	1 cup

Day 21

Breakfast

	1,200	*1,500*	*1,700*
• Bagel (preferably whole wheat, oat bran or other whole grain) with:	½	1	1
butter or margarine	1 tsp.	2 tsp.	2 tsp.
or			
cream cheese	1 Tbsp.	2 Tbsp.	2 Tbsp.
• Skim milk	8 oz.	8 oz.	8 oz.
• Orange-pineapple juice	6 oz.	8 oz.	8 oz.
• Peach	1	1	1

Lunch

	1,200	*1,500*	*1,700*
• Hamburger (3 oz. cooked)	1	1	1
or			
Vegetable burger, baked (p. 252)	1 patty	1 patty	1 large patty
with bun (preferably whole wheat)	1	1	1
ketchup and mustard	to taste	to taste	to taste
• Green salad 🔲 with:	1½ cups	1½ cups	1½ cups
regular salad dressing (p. 247)	2 tsp.	2 tsp.	1 Tbsp.
or			
reduced-calorie salad dressing (p. 245)	1 Tbsp.	1 Tbsp.	1 Tbsp.
• Apple or pear	1	1	1

Dinner

	1,200	*1,500*	*1,700*
• Yam (sweet potato) or potato, baked	1 small	1 med.	1 large
with sour cream (preferably reduced-fat)	1 Tbsp.	1½ Tbsp.	2 Tbsp.

(continued)

Week 3–Continued

	1,200	1,500	1,700

Day 21–Continued

Dinner–Continued

	1,200	1,500	1,700
• Broccoli, steamed, with spritz of lemon (p. 201)	1½ cups	1½ cups	1½ cups
• Strawberries (fresh or frozen, unsweetened) (p. 234)	1 cup	1 cup	1 cup

Snack

	1,200	1,500	1,700
• Graham cracker (preferably whole wheat)	none	none	1 whole rectangle
with jam	none	none	1 tsp.
• Skim milk	none	none	4 oz.

Week 4

Day 22

Breakfast

	1,200	1,500	1,700
• Bran cereal (p. 213)	1 oz.	1.5 oz.	1.5 oz.
with: skim milk	8 oz.	8 oz.	8 oz.
banana	1	1	1
• Orange juice	6 oz.	8 oz.	8 oz.

Lunch

	1,200	1,500	1,700
• Split pea or lentil soup (p. 250)	1 cup	1½ cups	2 cups
• Whole wheat bread (p. 210)	1 slice	2 slices	2 slices
• Tomato-cucumber salad	1 cup	1 cup	1 cup

Snack

	1,200	1,500	1,700
• Nonfat fruit yogurt (p. 253)	8 oz.	8 oz.	8 oz.

Dinner

	1,200	1,500	1,700
• Pasta with tomato sauce made with:			

	1,200	1,500	1,700
pasta (preferably whole wheat) (p. 239)	1 cup	1 cup	1½ cups
meatless tomato sauce (p. 240)	¼ cup	¼ cup	⅓ cup
Parmesan cheese	1 Tbsp.	1 Tbsp.	1 Tbsp.
• Brussels sprouts or cauliflower or broccoli florets, steamed, with spritz of lemon (p. 201)	½ cup	½ cup	½ cup
• Orange	1	1	1

Day 23

Breakfast ___

• English muffin (preferably whole wheat), toasted (p. 211)	1	1	1
with jam	2 tsp.	2 tsp.	2 tsp.
• Skim milk	8 oz.	8 oz.	8 oz.
• Orange juice	6 oz.	6 oz.	6 oz.
• Cantaloupe	½	½	½
or			
Mango	1	1	1

Lunch ___

• Vegetarian pizza	1 slice	1 slice	1 slice
• Apple or pear	1	1	1

Dinner ___

• Vegetarian beans (p. 206) Ɩ or vegetarian chili (p. 236)	¾ cup	1 cup	1¼ cups
• Brown rice, cooked (p. 243) Ɩ	1 cup	1 cup	1 cup
• Green salad Ɩ with:	1 cup	1 cup	1 cup
regular salad dressing (p. 247)	2 tsp.	2 tsp.	1 Tbsp.
or			

(continued)

Week 4—Continued

Day 23—Continued

Dinner—Continued

	1,200	1,500	1,700
reduced-calorie salad dressing (p. 245)	1 Tbsp.	1 Tbsp.	1 Tbsp.
• Plum or peach	1	1	1

Snack

• Cookie (2-in. diameter)	1	1	2
• Skim milk	none	none	4 oz.

Day 24

Breakfast

• Egg, poached or boiled	1	2	2
• Whole wheat toast (p. 210)	1 slice	2 slices	2 slices
• Orange juice	6 oz.	8 oz.	8 oz.
• Grapefruit	½	½	½

Lunch

• Peanut butter and jelly sandwich made with:			
peanut butter	1 Tbsp.	2 Tbsp.	2 Tbsp.
jelly	2 tsp.	1 Tbsp.	1 Tbsp.
whole wheat bread (p. 210)	2 slices	2 slices	2 slices
• Skim milk	8 oz.	8 oz.	8 oz.

Dinner

• Stir-fried vegetables and rice made with:			
stir-fry vegetables (p. 252)	6–10 oz. pkg.	6–10 oz. pkg.	6–10 oz. pkg.
brown rice, cooked (p. 243)	1 cup	1 cup	1½ cups
• Frozen yogurt or ice milk (p. 231)	¾ cup	¾ cup	1 cup
with berries (p. 234)	½ cup	½ cup	½ cup

Day 25

Breakfast

	1,200	1,500	1,700
• Bran cereal (p. 213) with:	1 oz.	1.5 oz.	1.5 oz.
skim milk	8 oz.	8 oz.	8 oz.
banana	½	1	1
or			
peach	1	1	1
• Orange-pineapple juice	6 oz.	6 oz.	8 oz.

Snack

	1,200	1,500	1,700
• Vanilla or lemon nonfat yogurt (p. 253)	4 oz.	8 oz.	8 oz.

Lunch

	1,200	1,500	1,700
• Lentil soup (p. 250)	1 cup	1½ cups	2 cups
• Whole wheat pita (p. 212)	1 mini	1 regular	1 regular
• Plum	2	2	2
or			
Grapes	15	15	15

Dinner

	1,200	1,500	1,700
• Pasta with seafood frozen entrée (260–300 calories) (p. 249)	1	1	1
• Asparagus spears, steamed, with spritz of lemon (p. 201)	7	7	7
• Whole wheat bread (p. 210)	2 slices	2 slices	3 slices
with butter or margarine	1 tsp.	1 tsp.	1 tsp.
• Fruit salad	1½ cups	1½ cups	1½ cups

Day 26

Breakfast

	1,200	1,500	1,700
• Bran muffin (p. 238) (avoid "jumbo" muffins)	1 small	1 small	2 small or 1 med.

(continued)

——— *CALORIES* ———

	1,200	1,500	1,700

Day 26—Continued

Breakfast–Continued

• Skim milk	8 oz.	8 oz.	8 oz.
• Orange juice	6 oz.	8 oz.	8 oz.
• Nectarine	1	1	1

Lunch

• Turkey sandwich made with:			
turkey breast (p. 227)	2 oz.	2 oz.	3 oz.
mustard	to taste	to taste	to taste
mayonnaise	1 tsp.	1 tsp.	1 tsp.
lettuce and tomato	as desired	as desired	as desired
whole wheat bread (p. 210)	2 slices	2 slices	2 slices
• Carrot and celery sticks	4 to 8	4 to 8	4 to 8

Snack

• Cookie (2-in. diameter)	1	1	2
• Skim milk	8 oz.	8 oz.	8 oz.

Dinner

• Lentil-rice pilaf from mix (p. 245)	1¼ cups	1¾ cups	1¾ cups
• Green salad with:	1½ cups	1½ cups	1½ cups
regular salad dressing (p. 247)	2 tsp.	2 tsp.	1 Tbsp.
or			
reduced-calorie salad dressing (p. 245)	1 Tbsp.	1 Tbsp.	1 Tbsp.
• Cantaloupe	½	½	½
with strawberries (p. 234)	5	5	5

| | CALORIES | | |
	1,200	*1,500*	*1,700*
Snack			
• Graham cracker (preferably whole wheat)	none	1 whole rectangle	1 whole rectangle
with jam	none	2 tsp.	2 tsp.
• Skim milk	none	4 oz.	4 oz.

Day 27

Breakfast

• Bran cereal (p. 213)	1 oz.	1.5 oz.	1.5 oz.
with:			
skim milk	8 oz.	8 oz.	8 oz.
banana	1	1	1
• Orange juice	6 oz.	8 oz.	8 oz.

Lunch

• Cottage cheese, 1% fat (p. 222)	½ cup	1 cup	1 cup
• Rye crackers (p. 229)	4	4	8
• Fruit salad	1 cup	1 cup	1 cup

Dinner

• Pasta with seafood frozen entrée (about 300 calories) (p. 249)	1	1	1
• Spinach and lettuce salad with:	1 cup	1 cup	1 cup
regular salad dressing (p. 247)	2 tsp.	2 tsp.	1 Tbsp.
or			
reduced-calorie salad dressing (p. 245)	1 Tbsp.	1 Tbsp.	1 Tbsp.
• Whole wheat bread (p. 210)	1 slice	2 slices	3 slices
• Frozen yogurt or ice milk (p. 231)	½ cup	¾ cup	1 cup
with strawberries (fresh or frozen, unsweetened) (p. 234)	½ cup	½ cup	1 cup

(continued)

	———— CALORIES ————		
	1,200	**1,500**	**1,700**

Day 28

Breakfast

• Whole wheat toast (p. 210) with:	2 slices	2 slices	2 slices
butter or margarine	1 tsp.	1 tsp.	1 tsp.
honey or jam	2 tsp.	2 tsp.	2 tsp.
• Skim milk	8 oz.	8 oz.	8 oz.
• Grapefruit juice	6 oz.	8 oz.	8 oz.

Snack

• Vanilla nonfat yogurt (p. 253)	8 oz.	8 oz.	8 oz.
• Banana	½	1	1

Lunch

• Lentil or split pea soup (p. 250)	1¼ cups	1½ cups	2 cups
• Whole wheat bread (p. 210)	1 slice	2 slices	2 slices
• Mango	1	1	1
or			
Cantaloupe	½	½	½

Dinner

• Chicken fajita (p. 238)	1	2	2
with tomato salsa (p. 235)	½ cup	½ cup	½ cup
• Green salad with:	2 cups	2 cups	2 cups
regular salad dressing (p. 247)	2 tsp.	2 tsp.	1 Tbsp.
or			
reduced-calorie salad dressing (p. 245)	1 Tbsp.	1 to 2 Tbsp.	1 to 2 Tbsp.
• Fruit ice or sorbet (p. 232)	½ cup	½ cup	½ cup

8

Mind over Matter: Controlling Overeating

You've just lost a fair amount of weight, perhaps with a little more to go. The past four weeks on the weight-loss regimen were fairly easy, even a relief, because with the 28-day menus there were no food decisions to make. But lately you've started going out more—the luncheon on Tuesday where the apple pie à la mode was too tempting to pass up, or the cookout on Friday night where that extra burger found its way to your plate. By Saturday, you stopped trying to eat light, thinking you'd blown it this week and resolving to begin again next week.

Sound familiar? Then you know how hard it is to stay on a calorie-controlled eating plan. Losing weight is easier than keeping it off. You've "been good," scrupulously followed the weight-loss plan and finally reached a healthy weight. Now you want to rejoin the nondieting world, to go out and have some fun again. Yet like an obstacle course, tempting foods and hard-to-control eating situations spring up in your path, and once you've tripped up on a few high-calorie, fat-rich foods, you no longer can muster the resolve to stay on course. You begin to lose heart.

By now most of you, especially seasoned dieters, *know* that ice cream, potato chips, nuts, hamburgers and chocolate cake are high in fat and calories. It's just a question of how to gain *control* over these foods so that you won't become another weight loss/weight gain statistic.

This chapter is really not about food or nutrition. All the nutrition *knowledge* in the world won't help you if you don't control your eating *habits.* This chapter explores what's going on inside your head when you are around food. It's about breaking the chain of events that causes you to overeat. We'll give you new ways of approaching situations so that you have control over food, not the other way around.

As with most skills, practice makes perfect. After you've perfected these food-control techniques, you'll be able to handle any eating situation—whether you're at a party or restaurant, at home or simply stricken by an intense craving for chocolate. Before introducing these techniques, we'll give you an invaluable tool to help attack your weight problem at the roots, so that you can solve it for good. And we'll show you what to do with that nemesis of dieters—the scale.

Cutting calories is just part of the weight-loss success story. Studies show that you also must use some of the psychological and motivational strategies. For instance, in a 1989 University of Pennsylvania study, 36 percent of people who were given psychological strategies to cope with overeating had kept their weight off one year later, compared to only 5 percent of those who just went on a diet without psychological reinforcement. Unfortunately, that 5 percent figure isn't unusual, even in some of the most highly regarded weight-loss programs.

What Will Make This Time Different?

There is one weight-loss center that boasts a much higher success rate. At Structure House, a live-in program in Durham, North Carolina, a survey showed that 65 percent of clients had kept the weight off or lost even more five years after leaving the program. The key to their success is something we also believe is essential—the *food/schedule diary*. It takes a little work, but there's no question that the results are worth it.

So, before we launch into the arsenal of psychological weapons to combat overeating in any situation, we're going to set you up with the basic diary strategy. Besides the Bran Cocktail (page 30), the food/schedule diary is the Bran Plan's only other "must." Everywhere else we give you lots of options and leeway, but the diary is too important to miss.

A Bran Plan Must:
The Food/Schedule Diary

Most diet diaries are simply a record of everything you eat each day. This is a good tool, but we're taking it a step further, turning it into a powerful ally that will give you control over food instead of the other way around. As you can see from the sample excerpt from "Anne's" diary on page 126, the left side of the page is for *writing down a rough daily plan*. Include any important events, and plan every meal and snack in as much detail as possible. Do this in the morning or the night before.

Also, block out a time for exercise. Be realistic: Don't try to squeeze it in if you don't have time. That sets you up for failure. But making an "appointment" to exercise helps ensure that you won't skip it.

On the right side of the page *write down what really happened, including how you actually spent your time, what you ate, how you felt and how hungry you felt*. If reality corresponds with the plan, just make a check mark on the right side of the page. When things go differently, write them down.

The reason the diary gives you control over food is that *you* are dictating the terms—deciding in advance what you want to eat. *However, if you stray from the food part of the plan, don't think you've failed*. Think of your unplanned eating as a valuable lesson and try to figure out what made you go off the plan.

You'll be able to figure out what situations cause overeating. It might be a reaction to stress (Anne's upsetting conversation with her mother), or it might be simple hunger—maybe you didn't eat enough throughout the day and were hungry at night. When you spot a pattern, try to work on changing it. For instance, Anne realized that most

Sample Diary Page

Day: *Friday, 3/5/93*

Daily Food/ Schedule Plan (list time and event)	What I Really Ate and Did (list time and event and any emotions or degree of hunger)
8:00 a.m. Wake up	✓
8:30 Breakfast at home:	✓
2 slices of whole wheat toast with	
jelly	
Glass of skim milk	
Small glass of orange juice	
Coffee with skim milk	
9:15 Arrive at work	✓
Noon: Lunch in cafeteria:	After lunch, bought 2 Hershey's
Turkey breast on whole wheat bread	Kisses and ate them. Felt satisfied.
with mustard	
Seltzer water	
Fruit salad cup	
5:30 p.m. Leave work	Had to work late, missed workout;
6:00 Work out in gym	annoyed
7:30 Get home and make dinner:	✓
Whole wheat pasta with tomato sauce	
Mixed greens salad with vinaigrette	
Small cookie	
8:30–11:00 Read, watch the 10	*9:00* Mother called, conversation
o'clock news, clean the kitchen	upsetting
	9:30 Went to corner store, got ice
	cream, ate most of the pint.
11:15 Go to bed	✓

encounters with her mother ended by overeating, so she worked on improving the relationship with Mom. Keep this diary for at least two months. If you miss a day, just make sure you resume the next day. Keep the diary whether you're on the Bran Plan for Weight Loss or the Lifelong Bran Plan. Use it in conjunction with this chapter's coping tactics for situations that cause overeating.

What to Do about the Scale

Another important tool is the scale. Like the food/schedule diary, think of it as a way to keep you on track. If it doesn't indicate the number you were hoping for, don't feel like a failure. Just thank the scale for its gentle warning, and keep planning ahead in your diary.

That warning won't be so gentle, though, if you avoid the scale for weeks and your weight creeps back up. Getting on the scale once a week will catch a weight-gain problem in plenty of time while avoiding the obsessiveness and futility of daily weighings. Daily weighings prove nothing, because body weight can swing up and quickly back down simply due to changes in water weight. (Water weight is extra fluid that your body retains when you've overeaten or eaten a lot of salt, or for certain other health reasons).

Ideally, you should weigh yourself on the same day of the week, on the same scale, at about the same time, without wearing any clothing. If you're home, it's easy to weigh yourself without any clothing on, but if you're at the gym or some other place, make sure you weigh yourself with the same type of clothing on each time, and without shoes. Using the same scale is a good idea because scales can vary in accuracy. Keeping an accurate scale in the bathroom is usually very convenient.

If you find your weight is up by a pound or two, watch your food intake for the upcoming week. The increase may just be water weight. If you're still up and even increasing by the next week, then this is a good time to examine your food diary closely and see where you're overdoing it. If you can't seem to get things under control, you can always put some structure back into your diet plan by going on the Bran Plan for Weight Loss for a week or more and following it as strictly as possible.

Tricks to Keep You from Tripping Up

Think back to the moments when you've overeaten, binged or given up on trying to lose weight. What seems to be your weight-loss Achilles' heel, the types of situations that interfere with your weight-loss efforts? Your food/schedule diary will help pinpoint those situations. As you read on, you'll probably recognize one or more patterns that have botched up past weight-loss efforts. When you finish the chapter, review those situations that apply to you and try out some of the techniques for preventing overeating in those cases. Even if the strategy sounds a little strange, such as a two-minute deep-breathing relaxation break, give it a try (this one is particularly effective). You'll learn techniques that have helped our patients stay on course as well as those proven effective in large research studies.

Although we're emphasizing ways of keeping weight off once you've lost it—weight maintenance—the techniques you'll learn now will also come in handy for *losing* weight in the first place.

See if any of these obstacles to controlled eating sound familiar.

Social Eating

Whether it's a business dinner, a ladies' luncheon, Sunday afternoon football with the guys or one of countless other occasions to get together with others and eat, the same problem arises: how to limit the amount of food you eat, especially fat- and calorie-rich temptations.

General Tips for All Occasions

1. **Visualize victory.** If you had to give a speech in front of your colleagues or if you landed the lead role in a play, you wouldn't dream of giving a public performance without rehearsing. Right now, being in control of your social eating is even more important than a speech or an acting role—so it's even more crucial that you rehearse. Take a few minutes at home, in the restroom before you leave work or even while traveling, to do some relaxing breathing exercises. When you are relaxed, tell yourself that you *will* control your portion sizes and stick to a sensible eating plan at the upcoming meal.

In the relaxed state, rehearse your lines and your movements for the upcoming event. Imagine yourself sitting down to eat at the dinner party and taking reasonable portions, refusing seconds of high-fat items and enjoying the party. If you're going to a cocktail party, imagine yourself taking one or two appetizers, then saying "No thanks" to the waiter carrying the appetizer tray—and feeling pleased with yourself for displaying such willpower.

Look in the mirror and tell yourself you'd rather skip the fat than get fat. Imagine what you look like at a comfortable weight and size, and tell yourself that the momentary pleasure you get from a steak and fries is not worth the pain of becoming overweight. As someone once said about sex, "The pleasure is transitory, the cost ruinous and the position ridiculous." The same could be said for overeating!

2. Don't deprive yourself of a food you really want. Deprivation may set up dangerous bingeing. All evening you've been staring at the chocolate cake sitting at the end of the buffet table, but not taking a bite. When you get home, you head straight for the freezer and binge on chocolate ice cream instead. A better strategy: Rather than denying yourself the cake, plan on eating a small piece slowly, and then compensate by eating smaller portions of other foods and completely avoiding foods that you don't care about.

Also, don't fool yourself into thinking that filling up on carrot sticks will keep you from wanting the cake. It's better to eat *controlled portions of foods you really like* rather than forcing yourself to eat only "healthy foods." By allowing yourself a measured treat, you can reduce the temptation to eat uncontrolled amounts of unhealthy, fattening foods later. So relax, balance your intake and go home with a feeling of achievement. You probably won't be tempted to open the fridge for anything.

3. Don't go hungry. If you know you have a dinner party in the evening or a string of holiday parties to attend one week, eat light, but don't starve yourself. If you're ravenous when you arrive at a dinner or a party, you'll find it much harder to control your eating than if your hunger is partially satisfied before you arrive.

For instance, if you know you're going out for dinner, make breakfast and lunch a little lighter than usual and build up fat and calorie credit by eating the most nutritionally healthy foods. These meals are the time to pack in high-fiber bran cereals, grains, fruits and vegetables and nonfat milk products—foods you probably won't see at the dinner party. Save any dessert or other uncontrollable high-fat splurge for the dinner party.

These light meals will keep you fueled throughout the day, and if you are still very hungry before going out, have a piece of whole wheat toast and half a glass of orange juice or half a bowl of cereal and skim milk to take the edge off your hunger.

4. Take your time. A reporter once observed Nancy Reagan chewing a single grape 28 times. This might be a little extreme, but the point is worth making: Chew your food carefully and eat your meal slowly. There's a scientific reason for this. It takes about 20 minutes for the stomach to stretch, or distend. At that point, the vagus nerve is stimulated and sends a signal to the brain that registers "full." In that 20 minutes or so before feeling full, you could still have shoved in loads of food and calories. So during this time it's especially crucial to eat slowly and moderately.

Party without Guilt

We'd like to convince you that you can have just as much or more fun at a party while keeping food under control. For many of us, part of the fun of parties is abandoning the usual constraints—we flirt a little, dress sexier, eat more and drink more. But once you feel in control over your eating and drinking you'll enjoy parties even more. You must believe that it's possible to have fun at a party and not wake up the next morning pounds heavier. Here's the strategy.

1. On arrival, make an immediate food inspection and eating plan. Whether you are watching the Superbowl surrounded by friends, beer, chips, dips and other munchies, or at a 50-dish holiday buffet, survey the entire food selection before you eat a thing.

Then make your game plan, *deciding which foods you really want, whether they are low in fat and calories or not.* Determine whether you'll be satisfied by half portions of anything—like half a piece of quiche or half a serving of chocolate mousse. Then check to see if there are any lower-fat, lower-calorie items that you'd just as soon substitute for the higher-calorie items. For instance, if it's all the same to you whether you have pretzels (low in fat and calories) or peanuts (high in fat and calories), then stick to the pretzels.

Once you've decided which foods are most important to you and which you wouldn't mind taking a half-size portion of, decide *exactly how much of each food you'd like, and stick to your plan without fail.*

2. Chew the (proverbial) fat. Remember, get-togethers are not just for eating. They are for catching up with family or friends. So, after you've made your food plan, *socialize*, keeping your distance from tempting foods that you've decided are not part of your plan. Tell yourself you'd rather leave the party with a full heart than a full stomach.

At a buffet or cocktail party, remember to stand as far away from the food as possible. Keep your back to the food, keep your hands occupied with a seltzer or a diet soda and keep your mind occupied with engaging conversation. Of course you can't avoid seeing the food at a sit-down dinner. At the dining table stick with determination to your serving sizes, and talk, talk, talk—and, of course, listen!

3. Pace your drinks. In addition to donating calories, alcohol can undermine your best-laid eating plans in a more insidious way. The same way a few drinks loosen up social inhibitions (fine for certain situations), alcohol also loosens control over eating, destroying your carefully constructed party eating strategy.

Always wait until you've eaten something before drinking. Then decide in advance how many alcoholic drinks you'll have. Space drinks at least an hour apart, for a maximum of two, or occasionally three, drinks. Dilute drinks with seltzer water to lessen the amount of alcohol. For instance make yourself a wine spritzer (half wine, half sparkling water) or mix your gin and tonic with less gin than usual and more tonic. If you like the security of a drink in your hand, have sparkling water with a twist of lemon or lime, a diet soda or a fruit juice spritzer in between alcoholic drinks.

4. Take a break. Sometimes it's best to just cut out for a moment, especially while the trays of appetizers whiz by at their most fast and furious. Find a private sanctuary such as the restroom to take a break and strengthen your resolve. A good deterrent to putting more food in your mouth is to rinse out your mouth and pop a mint. (Women, apply some lipstick.) Take a minute or two for some relaxing breathing. Then go back in and talk to someone you really enjoy to get your mind off food. Then if you catch sight of that garlicky appetizer or messy dessert, maybe they won't seem quite as appealing.

5. Wear something snug. You know you're starting to overeat when your waistband gets tight. To take advantage of this warning signal, men could go to a dinner party with their belts buckled right on the waist. And women (if you feel comfortable), wear something snug. A quick glance in the mirror at yourself in a form-fitting outfit will remind you of the figure you want to keep.

In Control at the Restaurant

1. **Make a menu strategy.** No matter what type of restaurant you're in, and whether you're with the boss, a client or your best friends, take the time to examine the entire menu and order for both pleasure and health.

First see if there are any lower-fat items you really like—from appetizer to dessert. If one of the lower-fat items is appealing, then you're already ahead. However, *if you're going to splurge,* decide where you'll get the most pleasure for your calories, and *splurge on one course only.* For instance, if you decide to have the chocolate blackout cake for dessert, order a plain green salad (dressing on the side) instead of the salad with Roquefort dressing. Go for the broiled catch of the day instead of the spareribs.

You're not locked into ordering a main course. If you really love the appetizers, order more than one, and stop there—you don't have to order a main dish. Often you get a much more satisfying and interesting meal without the main course. For instance, you could order soup such as lentil or wonton (remember, creamed or bisque selections are usually very high in fat and calories), an appetizer such as salmon gravlax or even (occasionally) a small order of calamari, a salad and a light dessert (berries, sorbet) for about the same amount of calories as one main dish of rack of lamb, steak or fettucine Alfredo.

2. **Enlist the help of the waiter or waitress.** Ask if you can have meats, poultry or fish broiled instead of fried or sautéed. Ask if you can substitute lower-fat side dishes—for example, a steamed vegetable with lemon instead of french fries. Restaurants usually accommodate customers' health requests; it's no longer considered rude or unusual to ask.

Food Cravings or Emotional Eating

Your in-laws (and their three kids) are stopping over for dinner and spending the night. Or you just hung up the phone after a tense argument with a friend. Or it's 4:30 in the afternoon and your boss gave you an emergency project that's due by Federal Express's last pickup at 9:30 P.M. Your first thought? Chocolate.

Whether it's chocolate, chips and dip, Hostess cupcakes or other favorites, certain foods seem to soothe us when we're under stress. Most of us have certain foods we turn to in times of nervousness, sadness, fatigue, boredom or even elation.

These are our "comfort foods"—they make us feel better, and they are very hard to give up. Some researchers believe that eating these foods may even lead to a change in brain chemistry, producing brain chemicals that give us a temporary lift—rather like a drug. But most experts believe it's simply the comforting associations we have with these foods that make us feel better. Remember those chocolate chip cookies baking in the oven ready for when you finished your homework? Or the tinkle of the Good Humor truck heralding not only cones and 'sicles, but also the fun of running out to the curb with the other kids? When the pleasures and rewards of childhood come back to ease the pains of today, they become hazardous to your weight-loss effort.

It's not the piece of chocolate you have every afternoon that will put on the pounds. Food cravings can ruin your weight-loss or weight-maintenance efforts because that piece of chocolate can turn into an entire bar or bars of chocolate, or one cookie can become a whole box. Food cravings can turn into food binges of 1,000 calories or more.

The two intertwined strategies for getting cravings under control are finding healthier substitutes and reducing the cravings.

1. Find lower-fat/lower-calorie substitutes for craved foods. Sometimes it's not the pint of chocolate Häagen Dazs you crave, but something—*anything*—smooth, creamy, cool and chocolaty. One of the smoother fat-free frozen yogurts might suffice. So no matter what your particular craving, try and figure out which taste or texture you are really seeking and experiment until you hit upon a satisfying lower-calorie substitution. Even though you have found a lighter substitute, the calories will still add up if you do not control the portions, so buy *single servings*. For instance, buy a single cup of frozen yogurt instead of a pint. Or get two loose Hershey's Kisses from the store, not a whole bag.

2. Understanding your cravings. One of the most intelligent analyses of food cravings was made by Alan Marlatt, Ph.D., director of the Addictive Behaviors Research Center in Seattle and professor of psychology at the University of Washington. He suggests picturing a craving continuum beginning with a person with no cravings (very few of us) and ending with the addict. Most of us fall in between, where we have occasional cravings and give in to some of them. The addict is unable to resist cravings and starts associating them with various times of days or various social situations.

Just as the dogs in Pavlov's experiments were trained to associate the sound of a bell with the expectation of food, the environment starts sounding off more "bells" (being in the kitchen, driving past a doughnut shop, hearing the baby crying) that stimulate cravings. Dr. Marlatt likens addictive cravings to any other addiction. A food addict feels the same intense desire for and experiences the same deep pleasure from eating chocolate, for example, that the alcoholic feels for alcohol or the gambler feels for the rush of gambling. An obsession with food can be just as powerful as an obsession with gambling, alcohol or sex.

There are many psychological reasons for becoming addicted to alcohol or gambling or food—for instance, an attempt to fill an emotional or spiritual void. For that moment, when the person is on a "high" while gambling or eating, she feels alive and happy. But the comedown is usually quick, and then she feels even worse.

The way to get some perspective (and control) over your cravings is to see them as something external—outside yourself—not a substance that your body chemically has to have, says Dr. Marlatt. He calls the craving problem the PIG—Problem of Immediate Gratification. He advises, "Watch the PIG, see where it comes from and when it gets most obnoxious [meaning when and what stimulates your cravings]. Learn how to handle the PIG by substituting other activities or foods for the craved foods. The more you give in to your cravings, the larger the PIG becomes; the less you succumb to your cravings, the smaller the PIG becomes, until one day it disappears."

3. **Conquer your cravings by fooling the PIG.** Fool the Problem of Immediate Gratification by doing something else as soon as it (your craving) comes around. Do something that will roughly substitute for the pleasure of eating the craved food. Remember, the less you give in, the smaller the PIG will become, until it's gone for good! Here are some tried and true substitutes to consider.

• Call a friend.
• Take a walk.

- Go out and buy yourself a magazine, or something else that's inexpensive.
- Exercise vigorously—go out for a run or take an exercise class.
- Relax and/or meditate. Once you learn about relaxation and/or meditation, these become invaluable tools for warding off cravings.
- Substitute a low-calorie food—an ice-cold lemon seltzer, a hot herbal tea, a diet drink, air-popped popcorn, rice cakes, fat-free pretzels and the like.
- Take out the atlas and plan a dream vacation.
- Use this time to go to your coworker's office with all the project details you've been meaning to discuss.
- Do a crossword puzzle or play a computer game.
- Go out and buy bubble bath (to conquer one craving), scrub the tub (when the next craving strikes), take a bubble bath (to conquer the third craving).
- Take your dog for a walk (bypassing the candy vendor).
- Play with your kids.
- Play with your cat.
- Look at your body in the mirror and think about how good you'll look at the next social event if you don't give in to your cravings.

4. Conquer your cravings by giving in to them. Oscar Wilde used to say that the only way to overcome temptation is to give in to it. In the case of controlling eating habits, there actually is some truth to this remark. If you have to confront a forbidden list of foods every day, these foods could become obsessions that you're at high risk of succumbing to. Ironically, one way of conquering cravings is by giving into them *in a controlled way.*

Besides all the psychological origins for food cravings that we've discussed, another underlying cause is deprivation. See if this sounds familiar: You go on a diet and decide that ice cream, chocolate, french fries and a host of your other favorite high-fat foods are now on the "forbidden" list. You steer clear of these foods for a few days, then you start yearning for them. In the supermarket you examine each carton of ice cream. You can't stop looking at the chocolate at the checkout counter. You pass your favorite fast-food joint and you can practically taste the fries.

By the end of the week you can't take it any more. You're at the supermarket and you buy a quart of ice cream, telling yourself you'll just have a few bites. But when you get home you polish off nearly the whole box in a few hours. Dieting and bingeing are often two sides of the same coin. Dieters binge and feel guilty, then the binger diets.

5. Reintroduce "forbidden" foods. We suggest taking most foods off the "forbidden" list and putting them back in your diet in a controlled, planned fashion. We say most foods because for some people certain foods trigger bingeing—and it's then very hard for them to stop. For some, that food is chocolate, for others it's chips or something else. The danger food may lead to bingeing on other foods. For instance, you've been careful to buy just one piece of chocolate, not a whole bar or box. But eating just the one piece of chocolate makes you crave more foods, so you keep opening the refrigerator door and nibbling on other foods—and before you know it, you've binged. *So, if you know you have certain danger foods, stay away from them.* By allowing yourself almost everything else, though, you shouldn't feel deprived.

The way you go about reintroducing "forbidden" foods is crucial—otherwise you may end up bingeing on them and gaining weight. The first step is to give your current diet some structure. Structure could help you put some of these "forbidden" foods back into your eating plan, and it will prevent you from getting too hungry and grabbing anything (like a box of cookies).

We've given you two good models for a structured diet—the first is the Bran Plan for Weight Loss, which consists of three meals and one or two snacks per day. Despite its structure, the weight-loss plan provides flexibility because you can eat these meals at the time most convenient to your schedule. Alternatively, use the guide in the Lifelong Bran Plan for planning your diet.

Once you've put some structure in your eating plan, you can carefully reintroduce "forbidden" foods. Make sure to write them in your food/schedule diary. For instance, suppose today is Monday and you want ice cream. Make the rest of your day low in fat and calories to allow for the ice cream. You could have a low-fat breakfast of bran cereal, fruit and juice; for lunch, a low-fat turkey breast sandwich (without too much turkey) and a diet soda; and spaghetti with a meatless tomato sauce and salad for dinner. Then, if you still feel like having ice cream, go for one large scoop at your favorite ice cream parlor. Buy one scoop, not a pint to take home. *Always buy only one serving of high-calorie foods, never a bulk amount.* After all, you can't eat what you don't have in your kitchen.

When you decide to have that scoop of ice cream is really up to you. You could have it either after lunch, between lunch and dinner or after dinner. By waiting until the desire seems most intense, you'll be leaving some spontaneity to it. We guarantee that you'll end the day feeling good: You've enjoyed the ice cream, and you haven't blown your eating plan.

So you see that even when you take a food off the forbidden list you must handle it carefully, making sure it fits into your overall eating plan. The goal is to *normalize the food, so it no longer becomes an obsession*—just another routine food (that tastes great!).

Even with careful planning, having rich ice cream such as Häagen Dazs *every* day is risky. If you feel you can't live without high-risk foods, then alternate lower-calorie or smaller-size ex-forbidden foods with irresistible high-fat and high-calorie foods. For instance, Monday you had a large scoop of heavenly hash ice cream, so on Tuesday you should go to the store and buy five individual Hershey's Kisses (not a whole bag!). Limit the really high-calorie foods to no more than twice a week and moderate the portion sizes.

Dealing with Your Family

Your best-laid eating plans could be foiled when you return home to find a box of your favorite cookies, opened, on the kitchen counter or a carton of ice cream in the freezer. Family members who are not watching their weight may not realize how destructive their food habits are to you. With just a little coaching, however, those you live with can become invaluable supporters of your weight-loss effort.

1. **Prepare yourself for your family's reaction to the new eating plan.** Interesting things happen when one person in the family tries to improve eating habits. In many cases, others who have been wanting to improve their own join in. It just took someone *else* to buy all the right foods. Maybe your wife had been wanting to lose weight also but thought it was hopeless with you around, so now she'll join you.

Your daughter might finally tell you how worried she's been about your unhealthy eating habits and might even help you prepare the new meals. Your husband could have been hoping you'd lose some weight but kept waiting for the right moment to tell you. So he'll happily join you at dinnertime.

On the other hand, your mate may not be so thrilled about your new eating regimen, particularly if he or she sees you becoming slimmer and more attractive. Occasionally, mates feel threatened by their wives or husbands or boyfriends or girlfriends becoming more attractive and (this is even more daunting) increasingly confident. This confidence comes not only from looking more attractive but also from the powerful feeling that you're gaining control over an eating pattern that has historically gotten the better of you.

So the insecure mate may try to sabotage your diet efforts by suggesting going out for ice cream, urging you to have second helpings or bringing high-calorie foods into the house. Since this is often an unconscious reaction, the culprit will surely deny that there is an effort to impede your progress. And it may be hard for you to determine if this is a new tactic or just a continuation of old patterns of behavior. But if you suspect that your mate is consciously or unconsciously trying to undermine your efforts at eating better to lose or maintain weight, then you must do something about it.

Try to devise a way to stop this subversive behavior, because it could pose a real threat to your weight-loss effort. Your approach depends on the nature of your relationship. It's best to deal with the obvious problem first—the tempting foods. You could say, "I'm trying to lose some weight and develop new eating habits. Could you help me?" Then ask if your partner would mind eating those foods that are not on your daily plan in another room, or having an ice cream cone at the parlor instead of bringing a pint home. (See our suggestions below for keeping other family members' foods out of sight).

You can deal with the underlying problem—the insecurity, the fear of losing you as you become more attractive and confident—either directly or indirectly, using a less confrontational approach. You could try reassuring your partner of your love and commitment to the relationship. Say you want to look and feel healthier for his or her sake as well as your own, without even mentioning the diet sabotage. After a month or so, if this doesn't work, you could discuss the underlying problem by saying something like, "I've noticed that you've been offering me foods that I don't want. I've been letting you know that I don't want to be tempted by these foods. I'm wondering if you realize this." Sometimes just bringing this behavior to your mate's attention could be enough to make him or her recognize it for the first time. That may be enough to change the situation.

If this behavior persists, you may have to tell your mate that you suspect it's related to feelings of insecurity, and then reassure him or her that there is nothing to be insecure about. If this insecurity shows up in many other areas of your relationship and is making you unhappy, you may consider some joint counseling.

2. Let your family have their cake and eat it, too. While you can't expect your whole family to change all their eating habits along with you, you can expect them to show some courtesy and support, just as your son would expect you to turn down the television if he's doing his homework or your wife would expect you to take off muddy boots before walking across the carpet. *Never feel guilty about asking family members to help you in your healthy eating efforts. By helping you, they are helping themselves.* They will wind up with better food in the house and a healthier mom, dad, brother, sister, husband, wife, boyfriend or girlfriend. Just keep these points in mind.

Your new eating plan doesn't have to inconvenience family members. The few changes they ought to make will soon become automatic. They should not eat certain foods in your presence. Also, they should buy *single servings* of ice cream, cookies, chips and other snacks and not eat them in your presence. For instance, they could have a candy bar at work, a cookie on the walk home or a small bag of chips in the basement while listening to the stereo.

If you must buy foods for your kids that are not part of your eating plan, keep these foods out of sight. If you have small children who insist on certain foods that will tempt you (animal crackers, peanut butter) put all these foods in a closed cupboard. Use that cupboard *exclusively* for the kids' foods, taking out only their portions and then returning the food to the cupboard.

Older kids can also have their own cupboard. If you're a binger, give them a large lockable metal box in which to store their cookies and other goodies, and give *them* the key. This sounds a little extreme, but it's effective.

No Time to Cook

If you find that your schedule is too full for meal preparation, you must find quick take-out, frozen or deli items that fit into your food plan. One great resource is the Bran Plan for Weight Loss Take-Out Plan. Appendix B on page 205 gives tips for low-fat, lower-calorie take-out choices.

So that you don't end up grabbing any old meal when you get home, plan ahead. Think about what you'd like to eat and where to pick it up. That way you'll be prepared in advance to pass by the deli or the Mexican carry-out or the supermarket on your way home. If you have a little more time, you can add your own ingredients to the prepared food. For instance, adding broiled chicken breast strips (the poultry section of the supermarket may have them precut and marinated) or tofu to frozen mixed vegetables turns a vegetable side dish into a complete meal.

Too Much Time to Cook

Obviously, it's easier to lose weight if you're not around food all the time. But for people who are food obsessed, whose world revolves around cooking and eating, it's difficult to stay away from food. One individual comes to mind. He would have a healthy dinner that matched his dinner plan, but later pore over cookbooks until he just had to go out and buy groceries and prepare another meal. All too often he couldn't resist eating again—as a result, he couldn't lose weight. If you love to cook and love to be around food, you are at a greater risk of gaining back the weight you lose. *You must limit your contact with food.* If you are a chef or your job involves being around food, you can limit your contact with food on your off hours. The trend among the new generation of chefs is to be thin, not fat.

Food can and should still be an important part of your life. But you mustn't fool yourself into thinking that constantly reading cookbooks, making batches of brownies and browsing in gourmet stores isn't going to tempt you. Go ahead and fuel your creative cooking fires by using the low-fat, healthy recipes in appendix A on page 173, or invent your own based on these recipes or guidelines in chapter 10. But if you still have creative energy to spare, find another outlet besides food or cooking—art, writing, dancing, gardening or anything else that interests you.

No Time or Desire to Exercise

Even athletes sometimes hate to exercise. So for anyone who's out of shape—especially overweight and out of shape—it's hard to get motivated. Then there's the time problem—10- to 12-hour workdays leave little time or energy for exercise. But it's crucial. Lack of exercise is one of the leading causes of obesity in this country, even among children, and a major risk factor for heart disease. As stressed before, you have a much better chance of keeping weight off for good if you are active. These tips should help you get on the active weight-loss track.

1. Remember, exercise need not mean high-impact aerobics. As we've told you in chapters 5 and 6, exercise means at least a 20-minute walk, a half-hour of gardening, 15 minutes on a stationary bike or just about any other form of movement that gets your heart rate up and has you breathing hard for 15 minutes or more.

2. Sneak in exercise whenever possible. Let's just talk about walking for a while—it's free and convenient, it requires no expensive equipment and almost everyone can do it. During the course of a normal day, you might walk over two miles, even if you didn't take a planned "walk." Actually, you can plan for walking just as you plan your diet. Just take a look at your day and think of any opportunities for walking—even if it's just a walk up two flights of stairs.

Your only piece of mandatory equipment is a pair of comfortable shoes. Keep them handy at all times. Stow them in an office drawer, under your car seat or in your briefcase or bag. Wear them during your lunch break, while shopping and on your way to and from work, church or anywhere. You can slip your "good" shoes on again right before you enter the office, the church or the party. To see how you can dramatically increase your exercise without putting a foot inside a gym, compare the two routines in "Going That 'Extra Mile' for Health" on page 142.

Practice Makes Perfect

Don't be too hard on yourself if your first attempts at gaining control over your eating habits don't always work, and use any "slips" as instructive lessons. Never give up. Practice makes perfect, and gradually, you'll find yourself controlling food rather than finding that it still controls you.

Going That "Extra Mile" for Health

Take a look at how one of our patients, Mrs. Clements, dramatically increased her daily exercise without setting foot inside a gym. Over the course of a typical day, every step of the way, she had two options: the inactive, "convenient" approach (taking elevators, getting the parking place closest to the building) or the energetic option (taking the stairs, walking to lunch).

Mrs. Clements weighs 145 pounds. Remember, the more you weigh, the more calories you burn doing any exercise. Compare the mileage and calorie tallies on the inactive and active options.

8:00 A.M.

INACTIVE: She drives to work, parks in the company lot close to the entrance and takes the elevator up to her office. Total walking: 30 yards. Total calories burned: 3.

ACTIVE: She parks at the distant end of the parking lot and walks to her office building (100 yards, 10 calories). She walks up the five flights of stairs to the office (45 calories—stair-climbing uses up more calories than walking). Total walking: 100 yards plus up five flights of stairs. Total calories burned: 55.

9:30

INACTIVE: She takes the elevator to the company cafeteria for breakfast. Total walking: 10 yards. Total calories burned: 1.

ACTIVE: She walks down the three flights of stairs (21 calories) to the company cafeteria for breakfast, then walks back up to her office (27 calories). Total walking: up and down three flights of stairs. Total calories burned: 48.

1:00 P.M.

INACTIVE: She takes the elevator downstairs, goes to a lunch spot around the corner, eats lunch, then walks back to her office building and takes the elevator up. Total walking: 50 yards. Total calories burned: 5.

ACTIVE: She changes into walking shoes and walks down five flights of stairs (35 calories). She allows time to walk to and from the farthest lunch counter, ten blocks away (1 mile, 150 calories at a fast clip). She walks back upstairs (45 calories), bringing her lunch back to her desk (to make up for walking time). Total walking: 1 mile plus up and down five flights of stairs. Total calories burned: 230.

6:00

INACTIVE: She leaves her office, taking the elevator down. Then she gets in her car (parked near the building) and drives to the super-market on the way home, parking close to the entrance. Total walking: 50 yards. Total calories burned: 5.

ACTIVE: She takes the five flights of stairs down (35 calories) and walks to her car at the other end of the parking lot (100 yards, 10 calories). She stops at the supermarket on the way home, parking at the farthest end of the parking lot. She buys a minimum amount of groceries, so she can comfortably walk back to her car (200 yards back and forth, 20 calories). Total walking: five flights down and 300 yards. Total calories burned: 65.

7:00

She gets home and starts to prepare dinner for her family. Total walking: Just a few yards. Total calories burned: maybe 1.

8:30

INACTIVE: She helps her kids with homework, then watches TV. No walking.

ACTIVE: She walks for 20 minutes at a fast clip before helping the kids. Total walking: 1 mile. Total calories burned: 150.

Daily Total

INACTIVE TOTAL: Minimum walking: 153 yards. That's 15 calories burned from walking. (Fortunately, we burn calories all day long just by existing, otherwise, we'd all be in worse trouble!)

ACTIVE TOTAL: Squeezing in the walking: a little more than 2 miles plus 13 flights up stairs and 13 flights down stairs. That's 548 calories burned (the stair-climbing made this total much higher than if those miles were accumulated by walking only).

At this rate, Mrs. Clements could lose a pound a week through exercise alone. Do you still think you're too busy to exercise?

9

Longevity
Nutrients
on the Bran Plan

*B*y now, you know that eating less fat and more fiber helps ward off killer diseases and keep you trim and energetic. And there's an added plus to this type of diet: Your vitamin and mineral intake shoots way up.

Switching to a low-fat, high-fiber diet is like taking a vitamin and mineral pill, because your new staples—grains, vegetables and fruits—are chock-full of nutrients.

This chapter will give you general guidelines for healthy eating. The next chapter will show you how to fine-tune your lifelong eating style for the ideal mix of foods from various food groups at your selected calorie level.

So, read on to get a general idea of what your new "balanced diet" looks like. You'll also learn about some of the "longevity foods" that are generating excitement in the nutrition community because of their disease-fighting qualities.

What Does a Healthy Diet Look Like?

Here's a very simple way to start thinking about how you should fill up your plate.

A healthy diet is just about the reverse of the typical American diet. Nowadays, about two-thirds of our foods are derived from animals (beef, poultry, fish and dairy) and about one-third are plant-based (fruit, vegetable, bread, grain and cereal). A good way to change to a healthier way of eating is to reverse the ratio to one-third animal-based and two-thirds plant-based. Picture your dinner plate with a small piece of meat, fish or poultry acting as a side dish and grains, potatoes, beans or vegetables taking up most of the plate.

Will a Plant-Based Diet Supply Enough Protein?

Animal-based foods are usually high in fat and cholesterol and low in fiber, whereas plant-based foods are usually low in fat and contain no cholesterol and are often fiber rich. But what about the protein supplied by animal foods? Isn't that very important? Actually, you need only 12 to 15 percent of your calories from protein. If you get too much, the body simply converts it to fat. And there's evidence that too much protein is linked with an increase in cancer risk. Only in poor third world countries is protein deficiency a problem. In the United States, most of us get way too much protein.

Contrary to what many people think, you don't need animal foods to get enough protein. Dried beans and grains will do the trick, usually with a lot less fat. But if you feel you can't do without beef or other animal foods, enjoy them in smaller portions, making them the side dish or using meat in kabobs, chili and so forth. Other good sources of protein are dairy foods, since there's as much protein in a glass of milk as in an ounce of beef. Stick to skim milk and other nonfat dairy foods.

In the next chapter we will show you just how many servings of animal-based foods can still fit into a healthy diet. But you can start thinking on the right track by giving plant-based foods center stage and downplaying animal-based foods.

Packing in the Nutrients

Why should you try to eat this plant-based, nutrient-rich diet when you can get all the vitamins and minerals you need in one or two vitamin and mineral tablets? The answer is that there are nutrients in foods we haven't even discovered yet, some of which may be critically important in the fight against all sorts of diseases. Every few months a scientist discovers another health-promoting compound in oranges, carrots, garlic or another food.

So that's reason number one: Eat healthy foods for the nutrients you *can't* get from tablets. Another reason is that getting your nutrients through a healthy, varied diet is a more natural, balanced way to get vitamins and minerals. High-dose tablets often give you too much of one nutrient at once. If a single nutrient dominates, it may prevent other nutrients from being absorbed. For instance, iron, zinc and calcium compete for absorption into your system. If you take high-dose supplements of these minerals at the same time, several times the Recommended Dietary Allowance, or RDA), the iron may block the zinc from being properly absorbed. When you take in small amounts of iron, zinc and calcium throughout the day in beans, cereals, grains, dairy and other foods, it's easier for the body to absorb these reasonable quantities without the problem of competition for absorption.

One final reason for getting your nutrients through your diet is that many nutrient-rich foods are often great sources of fiber while being low in calories—giving you a complete, well-rounded "packaged deal." Despite all these reasons, there may be a reasonable case for careful supplementation.

Should You Take Supplements?

Vitamins and minerals are crucial to our survival. Our bodies cannot make them, so we need to get them from food or supplements. A complete absence of these essential nutrients can lead to severe health problems and eventually death. If we had had any serious deficiency in childhood, we might not have survived to become adults. If we had any serious deficiencies in adulthood, we would get diseases like scurvy (a vitamin-C deficiency) and pellagra (a deficiency of niacin, a B vitamin).

Actually, the modern understanding of vitamins began in the eighteenth century with the observation that scurvy, which appeared in sailors on long voyages, could be prevented by giving them two oranges and a lemon every day. However, the world had to wait until 1932 for scientists to discover that the vital ingredient was vitamin C.

In contrast, the cure for night blindness that is caused by vitamin-A deficiency has been known for thousands of years. In 1500 B.C. the Egyptians recommended eating roast ox liver or the liver of black roosters to cure it. This was followed in ancient Greece by Hippocrates' suggestion that raw ox liver could be used to treat night blindness. Of course, no one at that time knew what was in the liver that was so important.

These examples illustrate a very important point: The history of our discovery of vitamins created a widespread belief that we must follow a diet that provides enough of these vital substances to avoid developing potentially fatal *deficiency diseases*—and that's all. That's why the National Academy of Sciences set up the Recommended Dietary Allowances, levels of vitamin and mineral intake that ensure that we don't get deficiency diseases. But over the past few decades, researchers have been looking beyond the deficiency-preventive aspects of nutrients to how higher doses of these nutrients can stave off cancer and heart disease, boost our immunity, postpone the effects of aging and extend and enrich our quality of life.

Many studies are in progress that will help to provide the proof needed to convince scientists that we should take certain supplements of vitamins and minerals to avoid disease, but this could take many years. Can we afford to wait that long? Is there any risk in taking certain vitamins and minerals in doses that are higher than we could ever get from our diets? The answer is sometimes "yes."

While we don't want to suggest that everyone should take supplements, many of you probably already do. In this event, be sure you use the supplements that make the most sense: those that are likely to give you the best defense against disease, in doses that are safe. After all, while waiting for the scientific results to come in, you might as well use the vitamins and minerals that research scientists have selected as the most likely to produce good results. Before we look at what these are, you should know that when it comes to vitamins and minerals, *more is not necessarily better*. Some fat-soluble vitamins like A, D, E and K are stored in body fat, and high doses can become toxic. Vitamin B_6 and niacin, although water-soluble, can also cause toxicity in large amounts, so do be careful.

As a guide to what you could take if you choose to, let's first look at the vitamins and minerals that protect against cancer.

Vitamin A and Beta-Carotene

Vitamin A is necessary for healthy eyes and healthy cells. The vitamin A in our foods comes in two forms and from two types of sources. The first form is the vitamin A that comes from animal products such as butter, liver, dairy products, meat, etc. The other form, beta-carotene, comes from plant sources. This is partly converted into vitamin A in the body.

As with so many nutrients, the goal with vitamin A is to get neither too little nor too much. For example, animals deprived of vitamin A will eventually die. People who consume large amounts of vitamin A for long periods of time develop symptoms of fatigue, lethargy, bone pain, throbbing headaches, sleeplessness, loss of body hair, dry skin and even emotional problems. None of this toxicity occurs when vitamin A is taken in the form of beta-carotene. When a molecule of beta-carotene is broken in half inside the body, it forms two molecules of vitamin A.

But in a very clever way, the body only permits this to happen safely. When enough vitamin A has been formed, the rest of the beta-carotene remains unchanged. But both beta-carotene and vitamin A are very important, so what this means is that the best way to take vitamin A supplements is in the form of beta-carotene. Major scientific studies presently under way suggest that supplements of beta-carotene will reduce the risk of some cancers and heart disease.

Suggested daily intake: 15 milligrams

Rich sources: Fruits (especially apricots, cantaloupes, mangoes, peaches and prunes), vegetables (especially those with orange flesh or dark, leafy greens such as carrots, broccoli, brussels sprouts, endive, lettuce, parsley, spinach and yellow and orange squash), fortified cereals and wheat bran. Liver, cod-liver oil, eggs and some cheeses are rich in vitamin A, but watch out—they're also high in fat and cholesterol.

The B Vitamins

The group of B vitamins includes thiamine (B_1), riboflavin (B_2), niacin, pantothenic acid, pyridoxine (B_6), B_{12}, folacin (folic acid), biotin and choline.

So far, there is no good reason to increase your intake of most B vitamins much above the RDA, which should easily be provided by the Lifelong Bran Plan. However, if you take a typical standard-strength multivitamin and mineral supplement, this will provide the RDA amount on top of your dietary intake. Although some studies are looking at increased amounts of folic acid to reduce cervical cancer risk and increased amounts of niacin to lower blood cholesterol, these examples should not be followed without consulting your personal physician.

Suggested daily intake: RDA levels (standard-dose multivitamin supplement). Women of childbearing age need 400 micrograms of folacin.

Rich sources: whole grain breads and cereals, bran (including the Bran Cocktail, page 31), pasta, fish, poultry, lima beans and some fruits and vegetables.

Vitamin C

Vitamin-C deficiency—scurvy—takes about three months to appear, producing extreme weakness, bleeding gums, joint pain and diarrhea and eventually leading to death. Scurvy can easily be prevented, however, by as little as 10 milligrams per day of vitamin C, which indicates how powerful such a small amount can be. Yet, large amounts in the range of 5,000 to 20,000 milligrams (5 to 20 grams) do not seem to present much risk. Excessive vitamin C can lead to diarrhea and occasional kidney stones. So far, there are no scientific studies that provide any reason to take more than about 500 milligrams per day. If you do take supplements for a long time, stopping them abruptly can also lead to some signs of scurvy, even when you continue to get normal amounts of vitamin C from your diet. So, be careful.

The possible benefits of taking supplements of vitamin C include boosted immunity, increased production of collagen, which improves wound healing, and even a lower risk of cancer and heart disease.

Suggested daily intake: 500 milligrams (slow-release supplement)

Rich sources: Citrus fruits (oranges, grapefruits and lemons), papayas, mangoes, cantaloupes, strawberries, watermelon, broccoli, brussels sprouts, green peppers, spinach and tomatoes.

Vitamin D

An adequate amount of vitamin D is necessary for healthy bone growth. In the past, when vitamin-D deficiency was not uncommon, it would cause children to develop a disease called rickets, which is associated with bow legs and poor bone growth. Now that milk is fortified with vitamin D, rickets is rare in the United States.

Although there is no need to get more than the RDA of vitamin D, there is evidence that people whose vitamin D intake is adequate have a lower risk of colon cancer. Do not take more of this nutrient than is present in a standard-dose multivitamin supplement; it can be toxic.

Suggested daily intake: 5 micrograms

Rich sources: Skim milk, certain fish (salmon, sardines, herring) and sunlight (which causes the body to make vitamin D).

Vitamin E

Discovered in 1936, this vitamin was first recognized as a factor that was necessary to restore fertility to rats brought up on cow's milk! Vitamin E acts as an antioxidant. (See "Selenium.") There is no evidence that a deficiency in humans leads to any signs of disease. On the other hand, there is a real possibility that supplementary vitamin E, particularly when combined with selenium, may lower cancer and heart disease risk.

Suggested daily intake: Research hasn't yet established the best supplement dose for disease prevention, but 200 to 400 international units is reasonable.

Rich sources: Bran Cocktail (page 31), bran cereal, wheat germ, oatmeal and vegetable oils.

Calcium

This is an important mineral that strengthens bones during their growth and development, maintains the body's calcium balance and can slow down the division of cells in the colon that are thought to increase the risk of colon cancer. In some people, it also seems to play a role in regulating blood pressure. Calcium also binds to fat during digestion, which may contribute to a reduced absorption of any harmful fats that may have crept into your diet.

Suggested daily intake: 800 milligrams (divided among meals)

Rich sources: Low-fat dairy products; dark green, leafy vegetables such as spinach and broccoli; and seaweed.

Selenium

This is a trace element that, like vitamin A, beta-carotene, vitamin C and vitamin E, is part of a system in the body that increases our antioxidant defenses. Antioxidants neutralize free radicals, which are produced in the body in response to pollutants and normal body chemistry. Unchecked, these free radicals roam the body like terrorists, instigating tissue damage that can lead to cancer and heart disease. Some studies have shown that selenium increases the effectiveness of vitamin E. In fact, one study of a group of people in Finland showed that those whose blood levels of selenium and vitamin E were the lowest had 11 times the risk of cancer compared to those with the highest levels.

Suggested daily intake: A diet rich in the following foods will provide about 150 to 200 micrograms. Supplements should be used cautiously, if at all, since selenium at high doses can be quite toxic.

Rich sources: Grains (pasta, cereals, the Bran Cocktail [page 31], breads) are good sources, but the selenium content varies depending on the soil in which the grains are grown. Meat, poultry and fish also contain selenium.

Longevity Foods

Although all vitamins and minerals are important, some appear to be more important than others. We want you to know about the more recent research into the "longevity foods," which contain nutrients and compounds that help to protect us against the most common killer diseases. Some of these nutrients have familiar-sounding names like vitamin C or beta-carotene; others you've probably never heard of, like indoles and coumarins. And there's exciting research in the works on producing foods that are super sources of these cancer-fighting, immune-boosting compounds. Now you'll have extra incentive to drink a morning glass of O.J., or eat a carrot or any of the other foods rich in "longevity nutrients."

Here are some of the foods that are under investigation as nutrition powerhouses. Some researchers are still trying to identify all the health-promoting nutrients in these foods—while other researchers are developing "superfoods" that contain extra amounts of these protective nutrients.

Carrots. One of the richest sources of the orange pigment beta-carotene, a substance that the body can convert to vitamin A, is carrots. Beta-carotene acts as an antioxidant, negating cancer-causing free radicals, which are produced in the body in response to pollutants or other triggers. Studies show that people who get lung, throat and mouth cancers have much lower beta-carotene levels in their blood and in their diets than members of the same population without these cancers. The U.S. Department of Agriculture has developed a carrot with three times more beta-carotene than regular carrots, which should be coming on the market soon. In general, the deeper the orange color of a carrot, the more beta-carotene it has.

Garlic. Studies in India and China have shown that populations consuming more garlic have a lower risk of stomach cancer, and this has sparked the interest of American scientists. In another Indian study, heart attack patients who ate six to ten cloves of garlic daily had 66 percent fewer deaths in a given number of years than patients who didn't eat garlic. Animal research shows that garlic helps prevent breast and throat cancer, and in test-tube experiments at the University of California, Los Angeles, garlic is showing promise in fighting skin cancer. Other animal research shows that garlic helps lower cholesterol and may even help reverse the buildup of artery-blocking plaque.

The same sulfur-containing phytochemicals in garlic, onions and other members of the allium family that cause their strong smell are probably also responsible for their health benefits. The sulfur compounds act as antioxidants and also "thin" the blood, reducing the risk of blood clots.

Garlic's phytochemicals change form, depending upon whether the cloves are raw, cooked, powdered (as a dried spice) or aged, making garlic research a complex task. All forms seem to be beneficial. Robert Lin, Ph.D., a longtime garlic researcher and president of Nutrition International in Irvine, California, recommends a daily dose of one to two cloves, raw or cooked, or six to eight garlic capsules (found in drugstores and health food stores).

Oranges and orange juice. Loaded with vitamin C, oranges and their juice are also emerging as nutritional superstars. Vitamin C helps reduce the risk of cancer and possibly even heart disease by acting as an antioxidant. Oranges also contain a collection of other cancer-fighting compounds such as flavanoids and coumarins.

Soybeans. These beans are rich in isoflavones, compounds that have proven in animal research to be successful in fighting breast cancer. The hormone estrogen, though essential, is one of the promoters for breast cancer; isoflavones act as anti-estrogens, which can reduce some of the effects of estrogen on healthy breast cells.

"It's hypothesized that soybeans are *partly* responsible for the much lower rate of breast cancer in Japanese women compared to women in some Western countries," says Mark Messina, Ph.D., nutritionist at the National Cancer Institute. Japanese women have much higher levels of isoflavones in their urine than Western women, says Dr. Messina, probably because on average they eat about 23 pounds of tofu and tempeh annually, compared to only ½ pound eaten by the average American. Although we consume lots of soybean oil in this country, it contains no isoflavones.

Cruciferous vegetables. Numerous epidemiological studies (studies looking at the diet and disease patterns of large populations in their natural living situation, not in a laboratory) have linked cruciferous vegetables—brussels sprouts, cabbage, broccoli, cauliflower, kohlrabi and mustard greens—to a lower risk of colon, lung and breast cancer. Cruciferous vegetables hold promise in preventing hormone-dependent cancers such as breast cancer because these vegetables contain compounds that affect the way the body handles hormones, according to one theory.

These compounds also alter the metabolism of bile acids, the "digestive detergent" in the intestinal tract that is known to promote the development of colon cancer. And more recent research at Johns Hopkins University has identified compounds called isothiocyanates in broccoli, which are potent cancer-fighting nutrients.

You'll find all these protective, healing foods in the Bran Plan Recipes in appendix A on page 173: a wonderfully potent pasta dish with brussels sprouts, low-fat goat cheese and garlic, plus other dishes containing broccoli and other cruciferous vegetables; a carrot coleslaw and other carrot-containing salads. Plus, you should aim for a daily glass of orange juice or other juice, and you can substitute tofu for meat in our chicken stir-fry and other meat dishes.

10

The Lifelong Bran Plan

Y ou are about to embark upon the diet that our bodies were designed for. This is the ultimate, natural diet; the diet of the early humans. Great things happen when your body finally gets back to the diet it was made for: You can control your weight, look better and have much more energy than ever before.

But let's be realistic, you're not going to last on berries and Paleolithic plants. You have to like your Lifelong Bran Plan, or despite your best intentions, you won't follow it for very long. So, here's your chance to construct a healthy eating plan that you really like and will stick with.

The three-step plan is simple: First, choose one of four calorie levels to maintain, not lose, weight. Then go to the *adding phase*—that is, add certain foods to your regular diet. The last step is the *substitution phase*—you substitute low-fat foods for high-fat choices and replace foods devoid of fiber with high-fiber alternatives. We guide you to the right food choices and the ideal amounts and combinations of foods. You plug in the fruits, vegetables, breads, whole grains, oils, spreads and foods you really enjoy. No counting calories—just think in terms of food groups.

If you've just completed the Bran Plan for Weight Loss, then you've already had a taste of a low-fat, fiber-rich diet. This gives you a head-start on the Lifelong Bran Plan, which is even more nutrient-packed, and, better yet, gives you unlimited food choices. If, on the other hand, you're coming straight off a typical, unnatural American diet, it'll take you a little while to adapt.

The plan is based on an intake of about 20 grams of fat and 45 grams of protein per 1,000 calories; the rest is carbohydrates. And, of course, it's high in fiber.

Choosing Your Calorie Level

If you have completed the Bran Plan for Weight Loss or another calorie-controlled diet, you know at which calorie level you lost weight. As a general guide to maintaining your ideal weight, choose a calorie level *above* the one you used while losing weight. Usually, men should try the 1,800-calorie plan and women should try the 1,500-calorie plan.

Within a few days you should be able to tell whether the calorie level is right for you. If you often feel hungry, you should eat a little more, so move to the next level. If you feel too full, then cut back one level. Checking your weight once a week is also helpful.

See the number of servings you should aim for in each food group on page 156. (Serving sizes are described in the lists that follow.) Remember, this should be your daily average over the whole week. So, relax. If you don't have a vegetable on Monday, have a few more on Tuesday or Wednesday, and the same advice goes for the other foods. But especially at first, try to stay as close as possible to your daily plan. Try to avoid too many exceptions. In time, you'll instinctively balance the right number of servings.

It's a good idea to keep a record of the foods eaten for the first two weeks, no matter how good your eating habits. (See chapter 8 for suggestions on keeping a food diary.)

Daily Servings at Four Calorie Levels

Food Group	Servings			
	1,300 Calories	1,500 Calories	1,800 Calories	2,000 Calories
Fruits	4	4	5	6
Vegetables	3	3	4	4
Breads/grains/cereals	6	8	10	13
Dairy	2	2	2	2
Protein sources	1	1	1	1*
Fat	3	4	5	5

*Athletes or other people who work out intensely may need a *little* extra protein. In that case, add an extra ounce of meat/poultry/fish or another ½ cup legumes or tofu. If you'd like to limit yourself to 2,000 calories a day, drop one of the fat servings.

The Adding Phase

After selecting your calorie level, strive for the recommended number of servings from each food group. This combination of foods also supplies a healthy dose of vitamins, minerals, fiber and other longevity compounds to your diet. In the lists that follow, vitamin C–rich foods are marked with a †. The beta-carotene-rich foods are marked with a *.

Allow at least two weeks to complete the adding phase. You might start with fruit for the first three or four days, then move on to vegetables, then whole grain foods.

1. **Adding fruits and vegetables**. Add any fruit to bring yourself up to the prescribed amount. If, for instance, you're on the 1,500 calorie plan, and you're currently eating 3 fruits, you need to eat one more fruit per day. Similarly, add the necessary servings of vegetables to bring you up to 3 a day.

2. **Adding high-fiber breads, grains or cereals**. Look at the list of

breads/grains/cereals servings. On the 1,800 calorie plan, for instance, you're entitled to a generous 10 servings. Estimate how many you eat each day, and if you eat fewer than your quota, then bring yourself up to that amount by choosing high-fiber foods, marked with a symbol on the list. If you're already eating the prescribed number of servings, there's no need to change anything until you enter the substitution phase.

   3. Adding the Bran Cocktail. If you haven't already done so, take the fiber quiz on page 32. Your score will tell you how much Bran Cocktail to add.

A Handy Guide
to Serving Sizes

   Some people can eat a soup-size bowl of cereal for breakfast, others are satisfied with ½ cup. To standardize the diet plan and eliminate guesswork, refer to these lists of serving sizes of fruits, vegetables and breads/grains/cereals. Keep in mind, however, that unless you are watching your weight very carefully, you do not have to eat precisely ⅓ cup rice or drink exactly ½ cup orange juice or whatever. Another mouthful or so won't make much difference.

Fruits and Fruit Juices

   Unlike vegetables, fruits vary considerably in size and calorie content, so we've given specific serving sizes. In instances where half a fruit (such as a banana) equals 1 serving, eating the entire fruit counts as 2 fruit servings that day.

   Fruit is an important source of vitamins and minerals, particularly vitamin C, plentiful in oranges and grapefruit and their juices. Whenever possible, however, eat the whole fruit instead of relying on juice—you'll get more fiber. Orange-fleshed fruits, like cantaloupe, are also good sources of beta-carotene.

   Unless otherwise specified, *a serving of fruit equals 1 medium to small fruit or 1 cup.*

1 medium apple or 4 dried rings

½ cup applesauce

4 medium apricots or ½ cup canned or 7 dried halves†

½ banana

¾ cup blackberries†

¾ cup blueberries

⅓ cantaloupe (5" diameter) or 1 cup cubes†*

¼ casaba melon or 1 cup cubes†

12 cherries

2½ medium dried dates

2 raw figs or 1½ dried

½ grapefruit or ¾ cup segments†

15 grapes

1 guava†

⅛ medium honeydew or 1 cup cubes†

1 large kiwi†

½ small mango†*

Nectarine†

½ cup orange or grapefruit juice†

Orange†

½ papaya or 1 cup cubes†*

⅓ cup passion fruit juice†

Peach†

1 small pear

2 medium persimmons†

¾ cup pineapple or ⅓ cup canned († if fresh)

½ cup pineapple juice († if fortified with vitamin C)

2 plums

½ pomegranate

3 medium prunes

½ cup prune juice († if fortified with vitamin C)

2 tablespoons raisins

1 cup raspberries†

1 sapote†

1 starfruit (carambola)†

1¼ cups strawberries†

2 tangerines (2½" diameter)†*

1¼ cups watermelon cubes

†Vitamin C–rich
*Beta-carotene-rich

Vegetables and Vegetable Juices

Vegetables are good sources of vitamins, minerals and fiber and contain some protein. Dark green, leafy vegetables like spinach, kale, collard greens and broccoli are rich in beta-carotene, which helps to prevent certain types of cancer. Dark green romaine lettuce and watercress also contain some beta-carotene. Orange-fleshed vegetables, such as carrots and sweet red peppers are especially rich in beta-carotene. Try to include these as often as possible.

Brussels sprouts, broccoli, cauliflower and cabbage are called cruciferous vegetables; diets high in this family of vegetables have been linked to a reduced risk of cancer. Choose them as often as possible. They're featured in delicious recipes in appendix A on page 173.

Potatoes and other starchy vegetables are closer in composition to breads and grains, so you'll find them in the breads/grains/cereals food category.

A serving of vegetables generally equals 1 cup raw or ½ cup cooked, or ½ cup juice

½ medium artichoke

Asparagus*

Beans (green or wax)

Bean sprouts

Beets

Broccoli*

Brussels sprouts*

Cabbage

Carrots or carrot juice*

Cauliflower

Eggplant

Greens (beet, collard,
  dandelion, kale, mustard,
  turnip)*

Kohlrabi

Leeks

Lettuce (romaine and other dark
  lettuces)*

Mushrooms

Okra

Onions

Peas*

Peppers (green, red or other
  colors)*

Rutabagas

Seaweed (nori)*

Spinach*

Summer squash

1 large tomato

Tomato/vegetable juice*

Turnips

Watercress*

Zucchini

*Beta-carotene-rich

Breads/Grains/Cereals (Including Starchy Vegetables and Legumes)

Grains and cereals are mostly made up of complex carbohydrates and contain some protein. They make up the bulk of the Lifelong Bran Plan. Complex carbohydrates are also found in vegetables as well as legumes (beans, peas and lentils).

Whole grain breads, grains, cereals and legumes are good sources of fiber and many of the B vitamins. They also contain a sprinkling of minerals such as iron, zinc and much of our selenium. Orange-fleshed starchy vegetables such as sweet potatoes, yams, and butternut or acorn squash are rich in beta-carotene. Choose fiber-rich whole grain breads, grains and cereals; white bread, white rice and foods made with white flour are low in fiber. For an extra boost of fiber, add the Bran Cocktail (page 31) to grains, cereals and any foods you bake yourself, such as pancakes or muffins.

Fiber-rich starchy foods are marked with a ★. Legumes are also protein-rich and work as a meat substitute (see protein list on page 165).

A serving generally equals 1 slice of bread or ½ cup cereal, grains or pasta.

Breads

½ bagel, 1 oz.(★ if 100% whole wheat)

2 breadsticks, crisp (approx. 4" × ½")

1 cup low-fat croutons

½ English muffin (★ if 100% whole wheat)

½ frankfurter roll or hamburger bun

1 pita, 3" diameter (★ if 100% whole wheat)

1 slice raisin bread (★ if 100% whole wheat)

1 small roll (★ if 100% whole wheat)

1 slice rye or pumpernickel bread

1 slice white bread (including French and Italian)

1 slice 100% whole wheat or multi-grain bread★

1 tortilla (not fried), 6" diameter (★ if whole wheat)

Crackers/Snacks

8 animal crackers

1½ graham cracker rectangles (★ if 100% whole wheat)

¾ matzo (★ if 100% whole wheat)

5 slices melba toast

24 oyster crackers

3 cups air-popped popcorn★

¾ ounce pretzels

2 full-size or 5 mini rice cakes, any flavor, no fat added

¾ oz. rye-crisp crackers (no fat added, such as Finn Crisps or Wasa)

6 saltines

¾ oz. whole wheat crackers (no fat added, such as Finn Crisps, Kavli or Wasa)

Grains/Cereals/Pastas

½ cup barley (★ if unhulled)

½ cup bulgur, cooked

½ cup couscous (★ if whole wheat

½ cup grits, cooked

⅓ cup rice, cooked (★ if brown)

3 tablespoons wheat germ★

⅓ cup bran cereal, concentrated (such as All-Bran or Bran Buds)★

½ cup bran cereal, flaked (such as Raisin Bran or 40% Bran Flakes)★

½ cup hot cereal, cooked (★ if whole grain variety, such as oatmeal, oat bran, multi-grain and whole wheat)

3 tablespoons Grape-Nuts

1½ cups puffed cereal (★ if whole grain, like Kashi)

¾ cup ready-to-eat cereal, unsweetened (such as corn flakes)

½ cup shredded wheat★

½ cup pasta, cooked (★ if whole wheat)

Starchy Vegetables

½ cup corn or 1 corn-on-the-cob, 6" long★

½ cup lima beans★

½ cup green peas, canned or frozen★

½ cup sliced plantain, steamed★

1 small potato, 3 oz., baked, or ½ cup mashed (no butter or cream)

1 cup winter squash, cooked (such as acorn or butternut)★

½ large sweet potato, cooked, or ⅓ cup mashed

Dried Beans/Peas/Lentils

⅓ cup dried beans and dried peas, cooked (such as kidney, white, split, black-eyed and chick-pea)★

⅓ cup lentils, cooked★

¼ cup baked beans★

Higher-Fat Breads/Grains/Cereals

These grain/cereal foods are higher in fat than those listed above. If you choose one of these, then you'll also use up one of your daily fat servings.

1 biscuit, 2½" diameter

2" cube cornbread

6 round, buttery crackers (such as Ritz)

10 french fried potatoes (2" to 3½" long)

1 small muffin (★ if whole wheat, bran or oat bran)

2 pancakes, 4" diameter (★ if whole wheat)

¼ cup stuffing, cooked

2 taco shells, 6"

1 waffle, 4½" square (★ if whole grain)

The Substitution Phase

The adding phase made your diet a whole lot healthier. The substitution phase will make it ideal as you strive to weed out or cut back on fatty foods and to complete the transition from low- to high-fiber foods that you began in the adding phase.

You'll make substitutions in the following food groups: dairy, meat/poultry/fish (and vegetarian equivalents) and fat (oil, dressings, snacks, spreads and so forth.) We'll even show you how to make desserts healthier. Then you'll re-evaluate your breads, grains and cereal choices and follow through on what you started in the adding phase—making all your servings low fat and fiber rich.

As with the adding phase, take the substitution phase one food group at a time. It's best to start with dairy for a week or two, then turn your attention to the other groups.

Remember, you don't have to eat anything you really don't like, just because it's healthier. Search for foods that fit your eating plan and also taste good. Keep experimenting—you'll find perfectly tasty substitutes either on these lists or among the new products on your supermarket shelf. Our brand-name guide will give you loads of ideas (see page 205).

Defatting Your Dairy Choices

Low-fat milk, cheese and yogurt are excellent sources of calcium. And low-fat or nonfat cheese can be considered part of the protein group because it can be interchanged, ounce for ounce, with meat, poultry or fish (see page 165).

A dairy serving equals 1 cup of:

Nonfat (skim) milk

½% milk

1% milk

Plain nonfat yogurt

Plain 1% yogurt

Note: If you customarily drink 2% or whole milk, try 1% until you get used to it. Then work your way down to nonfat (skim) milk. If you prefer to drink 2% or whole milk, each cup counts as 2 servings (for whole) or 1 serving (for 2%) of the fat group. (That's because 1 cup of whole milk contains 2 teaspoons of fat, and 1 cup of 2% milk contains 1 teaspoon of fat.) The same applies to yogurt—stick with the 1% or nonfat varieties.

A super-healthy snack is plain nonfat yogurt added to fresh fruit (and a touch of honey, if you like). This takes care of both a dairy and

Fat-Saving Dairy Choices

Instead of . . .	Fat (g)	Switch to . . .	Fat (g)	Fat Saved (g)
Whole milk, 1 cup	8	2% milk, 1 cup	5	3
2% milk, 1 cup	5	1% milk, 1 cup	3	2
1% milk, 1 cup	3	Skim milk, 1 cup	0	3
Whole milk yogurt, plain, 1 cup	7	Low-fat yogurt, plain, 1 cup	4	3
Low-fat yogurt, plain, 1 cup	4	Nonfat yogurt, plain, 1 cup	0	4
Low-fat fruit-flavored yogurt, 1 cup	3	Nonfat yogurt, plain 1 cup, with fresh fruit	0	3
Coffee cream, 1 tablespoon	3	2% milk, 1 tablespoon	trace	3

a fruit serving. However, if you're on the run or prefer the fruit-flavored yogurt, then you must count it as a dairy and a breads/grains/cereals serving. That's because the jam and sugar used to make it adds 80 to 100 calories, about the same as a serving from the breads/grains/cereals group.

Protein Sources

When you think of protein, don't just think meat. It's possible to get a perfectly adequate supply of protein from plant sources. True, there is no one plant food that contains as much protein as meat, ounce for ounce, but a diet that is dominated by vegetables, breads, grains, cereals, dried beans and/or tofu will provide more than enough protein. The classic combination, beans and rice, is a staple in many cultures. (Many people incorrectly assume that the more protein you eat, the better. Actually, eating too much protein can put undue strain on your kidneys or cause other health problems.)

If you are a vegetarian, or just enjoy a meat-free day once in a while (by meat, we mean beef, chicken, fish, etc.), the Lifelong Bran Plan enables you to choose between both animal- and plant-based sources of protein. The idea is to substitute foods from the "Low-Fat Meat/Poultry/Fish" and "Vegetarian Sources of Protein" lists below for foods you customarily select from the "High-Fat Protein Sources" list.

On the Lifelong Bran Plan *you are aiming for a daily total of 3 ounces (containing 8 grams of fat) of cooked meat, poultry, fish, shellfish or game (about the size of a deck of cards), or the vegetarian equivalent (tofu or beans).*

If you so choose, you may get your protein from a combination of vegetarian and meat sources. Let's say you had chicken fajitas for lunch, containing about 2 ounces chicken. Then for dinner, you get the rest of your protein from ½ cup beans.

Low-Fat Meat/Poultry/Fish

Lean beef (USDA Select or Choice grades, such as round, sirloin, flank steak, tenderloin and chipped beef)

Lean pork (such as fresh ham; canned, cured or boiled ham‡; Canadian bacon‡ and tenderloin)

Veal (except for veal cutlets; they are higher in fat)

Poultry, skin removed, *not* fried (such as chicken, turkey, ground *breast meat* turkey, Cornish hen, pheasant, wild duck and wild goose)

95% fat-free luncheon meat

Game (such as rabbit, venison or squirrel)

Fish, *not* fried (such as flounder, bass, salmon, etc.)

3 oz. tuna (¼ cup), canned in water

2 oz. lobster, crab, scallops, shrimp or clams

‡Cured meats, and unless labeled nitrite-free, may contain nitrites, additives linked with increased cancer risk. So eat them infrequently (no more than once or twice a month).

Vegetarian Sources of Protein

Here are low-fat vegetarian equivalents of low-fat meat/poultry/fish.

Cooked or canned beans (legumes): ½ cup = 1 ounce low-fat meat/poultry/fish *plus* 1 breads/grains/cereals serving (because legumes are rich in *both* protein and carbohydrate).

To get your entire day's protein from beans, eat 1½ cups, which also takes care of 3 breads/grains/cereals servings. Try kidney beans, lentils, white beans, black-eyed peas, black beans and split peas.

Low-fat cheese and egg equivalents: 1 ounce low-fat meat/poultry/fish = ¼ cup low-fat cottage cheese; 1 ounce fat-free or very low fat cheese, with no more than 55 calories per ounce, or 3 egg whites.

High-Fat Protein Sources

Note: These can hit you with up to 30 grams of fat per 3-ounce serving, so have these foods infrequently.

Beef (ground beef, including extra-lean; rib, chuck and rump roasts; cubed, Porterhouse and T-bone steak; ribs and most other USDA Prime cuts; corned beef; meatloaf and frankfurter‡)

Pork products (chops, loin roast, Boston butt, cutlets, spareribs, ground pork and pork sausage‡)

Lamb (chops, leg, roast or ground)

Poultry (chicken with skin; domestic duck or goose; ground turkey, except for all-breast meat; anything fried)

Fish (canned tuna or sardines in oil or canned salmon; anything fried)

Full-fat, regular cheese (Cheddar, brie, etc.)

Eggs: high in cholesterol; limit to one per week

Organ meats (liver, heart, kidney, etc.) also high in cholesterol; limit to once a week.

‡Cured meats, and unless labeled nitrite-free, may contain nitrites, additives linked with increased cancer risk. So eat them infrequently (no more than once or twice a month).

A Caveat about Two Vegetarian Staples

Tofu and peanut butter are high in fat, but unlike a fatty piece of meat or chicken with skin, these foods are low in artery-clogging saturated fat. So, if you like these foods, you can eat them daily, but just compensate for the extra fat somewhere else, by having a little less salad dressing, or cutting out another fatty food that day.

The following are equivalent in protein to an ounce of meat/poultry/fish.

4 oz. tofu (2½ × 1¾ × 1½" block)

1 tablespoon peanut butter

Choosing Carefully from the "Fat" Category

Generally speaking, a fat serving is 1 teaspoon oil or butter or other spreads; a tablespoon of nuts (yes, nuts derive about 80 percent of their calories from fat, so are classified as fats); a tablespoon of salad dressing; and 2 tablespoons of light cream.

A little bit of fat (like salad dressing) makes food more palatable and provides essential fatty acids, but too much fat (especially saturated fat) contributes to cancer and heart disease. So aim for selections on the "Rich in Unsaturated Fats" list, eat items on the "Nuts and Seeds" list sparingly and avoid selections on the "High in Saturated Fats" list (on page 168).

Fat-Saving Protein Choices

Lean doesn't have to mean tough. Lean meat or poultry without skin will be juicy if you cook it right. Marinate the meat or poultry and broil, bake or lightly stir-fry it until done, but no longer. Remember, for safety's sake, chicken and pork must be cooked all the way through.

Instead of . . .	Fat (g)	Eat . . .	Fat (g)	Fat Saved (g)
Beef, ribs or ground, 3 oz., broiled	18–26	Top loin or top sirloin, 3 oz., broiled	6–9	9–20
Beef, ground, extra-lean, 3 oz., broiled	14	Ground turkey, 3 oz., broiled	8	6
Beef hot dog	16	Healthy Choice hot dog	1	15
Beef potpie, frozen, 10 oz., cooked	31	Oriental beef frozen dinner, 10 oz., cooked	8	23
Beef, bean and cheese burrito	22	Bean burrito, no sour cream or cheese	5	17
Chili con carne, 1 cup	16	All-bean chili, 1 cup	4	12
Chicken breast, roasted, with skin, 3 oz.	7	Chicken breast, roasted, without skin, 3 oz.	3	4
Chicken drumstick, batter-dipped, fried	11	Chicken drumstick, roasted, without skin	2	9
Ground turkey, 3 oz., broiled	8	Ground turkey, breast only, 3 oz., broiled	1	7
Fish, breaded, fried, 3 oz.	12	Fish, in oil/lemon marinade, 3 oz.	4	8
Tuna, canned in oil, 3 oz.	7	Tuna, canned in water, 3 oz.	2	5
Mozzarella, whole milk, 1 oz.	6	Mozzarella, part skim, 1 oz.	5	1
Mozzarella, part skim, 1 oz.	5	Mozzarella, nonfat, 1 oz.	0	5
Cottage cheese, creamed (4%), ½ cup	5	Cottage cheese (1%), ½ cup	1	4

Here are the specifics. Everything on the following lists contains 5 grams of fat.

Rich in Unsaturated Fats

1 tablespoon diet margarine

1 teaspoon margarine

1 teaspoon regular mayonnaise

1 tablespoon reduced-calorie mayonnaise

2 teaspoons mayonnaise-type salad dressing

1 tablespoon reduced-calorie, mayonnaise-type salad dressing

2 tablespoons reduced-calorie salad dressing

1 tablespoon oil-type salad dressing (such as vinaigrette)

1 teaspoon vegetable oil (such as olive, canola, corn or safflower)

1 medium avocado

10 small or 5 large olives

6 almonds, whole, shelled

1 tablespoon cashews

1 tablespoon nuts, other varieties, shelled

20 small or 10 large peanuts

2 pecans, whole

1 tablespoon seeds (pine nuts or sunflower seeds), shelled

2 teaspoons pumpkin seeds, unshelled

2 walnuts, whole, shelled

High in Saturated Fats

1 teaspoon butter

1 slice bacon

1 tablespoon cream cheese

1 tablespoon heavy whipping cream (2 tablespoons whipped)

2 tablespoons light cream (coffee)

2 tablespoons shredded coconut

2 tablespoons liquid nondairy creamer

4 teaspoons powdered nondairy creamer

2 tablespoons sour cream

Substitutes for High-Fat Snacks, Dressings, Sauces and Spreads

Even small amounts of these foods are loaded with fat and calories, so small changes mean big fat savings.

Instead of . . .	Fat (g)	Eat . . .	Fat (g)	Fat Saved (g)
Broccoli with cheese sauce, ½ cup	12	Broccoli with lemon juice and herbs, ½ cup	0	12
Butter or margarine, 1 tablespoon	12	Butter or margarine, 1 teaspoon	4	8
Butter, stick, 1 tablespoon	12	Butter, whipped, 1 tablespoon	7	5
Margarine, regular, 1 teaspoon	4	Margarine, reduced-calorie, 1 teaspoon	2	2
Chinese take-out: stir-fried vegetables, 1 cup	5–15*	Chinese take-out: steamed vegetables, 1 cup	0	5–15*
French fries, 20	16	New potatoes, boiled, 3	0	16
Nuts, mixed, ½ cup	40	Trail mix, ½ cup	18	22
Peanuts, shelled, ½ cup	36	Pretzels, thin, 10	1	35
Pizza with everything, 1 slice	20	Pizza, single cheese, with vegetables, 1 slice	9	11
Popcorn, oil-popped or microwave, 3 cups	9	Popcorn, air-popped, 3 cups	0	9
Potato chips, 10	7	Popcorn, air-popped, 1 cup	0	7
Salad with 2 tablespoons Italian dressing	14	Salad with 2 teaspoons Italian dressing	5	9
Salad with 1 tablespoon Italian dressing	7	Salad with 1 tablespoon reduced-calorie Italian dressing (6 calories per tablespoon)	1	6
Vegetables, sautéed in butter, ½ cup	8	Vegetables, raw, 1 cup	0	8
Vegetables, stir-fried in 1 tablespoon oil	14	Vegetables, stir-fried in 1 teaspoon oil	5	9

*Varies from chef to chef

What Should You Do about Desserts and Snacks?

When your diet is basically sound, it won't be shaken by an occasional indulgence in a rich dessert or "junk food." Eating a little of these foods may even help; if you deprive yourself completely, you may end up bingeing on them later. Your strategy: Nothing is forbidden, just be moderate. For some of us, there are certain foods that are very difficult to eat in moderation, foods that trigger a major binge. So, if you can live without them, do so, and try to find satisfying substitutes. That means, for example, if chocolate bars are your weakness, try to be satisfied with a chocolate cookie. Reread the cravings section of chap-

Substitutes for High-Fat Desserts

If desserts are your weakness, this chart may help you wean yourself off slowly, by switching to sweets that are lower in fat and calories.

Instead of . . .	Fat (g)	Eat . . .	Fat (g)	Fat Saved (g)
Fruit pie with top and bottom crusts, 1 slice (⅙ of a 9″ pie)	18	Fruit tart with one crust, 1 slice (⅙ of a 9″ pie)	9	9
Ice cream, premium (gourmet type), ½ cup	18	Ice cream, regular (supermarket type), ½ cup	7	11
Ice cream, regular, ½ cup	7	Frozen yogurt, ½ cup	3	4
Pecan pie, 1 slice (⅙ of a 9″ pie)	32	Fruit tart with one crust, 1 slice (⅙ of a 9″ pie)	9	23
Two-layer sheet cake with icing, 2½″ square	12	Angel food cake with raspberry puree, 1/12 of a Bundt cake	0	12

ter 8, for other strategies to help you overcome your cravings.

Here is how rich desserts or junk food (like potato chips) fit into your food plan. First of all, unless you are satisfied with a tiny "homeopathic" dose, you cannot have this type of food too often. Once or twice a week is fine—you can either make up for it the same day, or you can eat a little lighter the next day. For instance, if you eat a piece of chocolate cake on top of all your other daily servings, then have less fat than usual the next day. Or, you can plan for the cake by passing up some other source of fat that day. Enjoy everything you eat, but just *be aware of what you're eating*.

Lower-Fat Breads, Grains and Cereals

Now that you have searched and destroyed (or replaced) high-fat dairy, meats, fats and fatty desserts, you have one last mission: defatting your breads/grains/cereals group. In the adding phase, you added on a few lower-fat items from the list on pages 160–61. Now, replace higher-fat items with lower-fat foods—a whole grain roll for a croissant, for example (also adding fiber). And remember, you can boost the fiber level of homemade baked goods by adding some of the Bran Cocktail. The table on page 172 should help.

Slow and Steady Wins in the Long Run

A handy way to add suggested foods to your diet or make healthy substitutions is to make a list of your preferred foods in each food group. Tack your mini-list on the fridge to remind yourself of all the healthy foods you can pick up at the supermarket, or the healthy dishes you can make for dinner.

Now, take the plunge into health. Start right now, by eating a fruit. Every time you make one meal lower in fat and higher in fiber, you've taken a big step toward a healthier, fuller life. Bon Appetit!

Substitutes for High-Fat Breads, Grains and Cereals

Grains are low in fat, but fat levels on baked products can soar because of butter, cream or oil called for in recipes. Same with pasta and bread: Topping your linguine with a rich, creamy sauce or smearing your bread with butter quickly turns a low-fat menu item into a high-fat food. So spread much less margarine or butter on your bread, and use low-fat pasta sauces (mostly meatless tomato sauces). Ask how sauces are prepared; anything with cream, butter or oil is high in fat. Sometimes, substituting another item doesn't lower your fat intake, but it boosts your fiber, making it the smarter alternative.

Instead of . . .	Fat (g)	Eat . . .	Fat (g)	Fat Saved (g)	Fiber Gained (g)
Biscuit, fast food	6	Whole wheat roll	2	4	2.0
Chocolate chip cookies, 2 (each: 0.5 oz., 2½" diameter)	4	Graham crackers, 2 (whole rectangles) with honey	0	4	0
Croissant	15	Whole grain roll	2	13	1.0
Doughnut, glazed	12	Whole wheat English muffin, with jelly	0	12	2.2
Graham cracker (whole rectangle)	0	Whole wheat or oat bran graham cracker	0	0	3.1
Granola, ½ cup	17	Bran cereal, like Kellogg's All-Bran, ½ cup	1	16	10.0
Muffin, large (4.5 oz. or 3" high)	9	Muffin, small (1.5 oz. or 1½" high)	3	6	0
Muffin, small	3	Bran muffin, small	3	0	2.5
Rice, fried, ½ cup	6	Rice, steamed, ½ cup	0	6	0
Rice, white, cooked, ½ cup	0	Rice, brown, cooked, ½ cup	0	0	1.0

A

Bran Plan Recipes

*I*n this section you will find the recipes referred to in chapter 7. If you're following the Bran Plan for Weight Loss, check your particular calorie level for the appropriate serving amount.

Except for the Bran Cocktail Muffins and a few other dishes that store well in the freezer or refrigerator, all these recipes make only one serving. You may, of course, multiply all the recipes to serve as many people as you'd like (in fact, most dishes are easier to cook that way). Keep in mind that if you're multiplying a stir-fry or a sauté, for instance, you can get away with using proportionately less oil; you don't have to multiply the oil by the same amount as the rest of the ingredients. Let's say you want to make a vegetable stir-fry for four people, and the single-serving recipe requires 1 teaspoon of oil for 2 cups of vegetables. You'll probably need only 2 or 3 teaspoons of oil to stir-fry the 8 cups of vegetables.

Note: Recipes that are suited to the Bran Cocktail (page 31) are marked with a 🥤. For every tablespoon of the Bran Cocktail you add while cooking, add 3 tablespoons of additional water or other liquid. Otherwise, you can just sprinkle the bran on top after cooking.

Equipment and Supplies

The recipes in this book are so easy and straightforward that you probably already have all the utensils you'll need. If you don't own the following items, however, consider them a worthwhile investment.

- A wok for all the stir-fried dishes (however, a heavy skillet will do)
- A colander to make washing vegetables and draining pasta easier
- A muffin pan
- A steamer (a folding metal insert that fits in almost any pot is sufficient)

Even if you're not planning on making all the recipes, stock up on the following basic ingredients that are essential for healthy cooking in general.

- Canola oil (great in stir-fries and muffins)
- Olive oil (for salads and sautés; seek out a flavorful brand that is satisfying even in small amounts)
- Fresh garlic
- Fresh lemons
- Italian or flat-leaf parsley (more flavorful than the common curly variety)
- Brown rice (especially the fragrant Basmati type)

Bean Dishes

You may use either dried or canned beans in these recipes. If you opt for the canned ones, which are certainly less work, you'll want to rinse them (unless the recipe says otherwise) to remove excess sodium and the thick liquid in which they're packed. Simply spoon the beans into a strainer and hold them under cold running water.

If you prefer to use dried beans, you'll have to soak most types before cooking. Lentils and split peas don't actually *need* soaking, but we feel even they benefit from the process. Here's what to do.

- Place the beans in a colander or sieve and rinse with cold water. Transfer to a large bowl and add four times as much cold water as beans. Regardless of what some recipes say, do not add baking soda during soaking or cooking because it will destroy certain nutrients.
- Soak the beans at room temperature all day or overnight. (Or take this shortcut: Rinse them as above and place in a pot with four times as much water. Bring to a boil and cook for 2 minutes.)
- Drain the beans, add fresh water and simmer until tender, 1¼ to 3 hours, depending on the type. Lentils and split peas cook quickest; white beans and chick-peas seem to take the longest. A recipe may require that you use the cooking liquid, so check the directions.

Note: 1 cup of dried beans, lentils or split peas expands to 2 to 2½ cups during cooking.

THICK LENTIL SOUP

This recipe might seem like it makes a lot, but it appears often in the weight-loss menu plans. Use what you need for the first meal, then freeze the remainder in portion-controlled containers.

8	cups water	1	onion, chopped
1¾	cups lentils or split peas	½	cup chopped celery
1	whole onion, peeled	1	teaspoon dried thyme
1	bay leaf	1	tablespoon olive oil
1	teaspoon salt		Chopped parsley or
1	large carrot, chopped		cilantro (coriander)

In a 3-quart saucepan over high heat, bring the water, lentils or split peas, whole onion, bay leaf and salt to a boil. Reduce the heat to medium-low and simmer, stirring occasionally, for 1 hour. Remove and discard the onion and bay leaf.

In a large frying pan over medium heat, sauté the carrots, chopped onions, celery and thyme in the oil for 5 minutes, or until the onions soften and turn golden. Stir into the soup. Simmer for 30 t0 40 minutes.

Ladle about 3 cups of soup into a blender and puree. Stir into the remaining soup. Serve garnished with parsley or cilantro.

Makes 9 cups
Per cup: 119 calories, <1 gram fat, 5.5 grams dietary fiber

TOMATO-BEAN STEW

This recipe makes two servings. If you're following the Bran Plan for Weight Loss menu plan, look for it on Days 3 and 23.

We like to prepare this recipe using white beans, such as navy beans or cannellini, but you may use chick-peas or any other type of bean. Serve the stew over rice.

1½ teaspoons olive oil	1 cup water or tomato juice
1 cup chopped onions	2 teaspoons dried thyme
1 can (15 ounces) white beans, rinsed and drained, or 2 cups cooked	1 bay leaf
	Salt and pepper (to taste)
1 cup coarsely chopped plum tomatoes (canned low-sodium or very ripe fresh)	

In a medium frying pan over medium-high heat, heat the oil. Add the onions and sauté, stirring frequently, for 3 minutes, or until they start to wilt and turn golden.

Stir in the beans, tomatoes, water or tomato juice, thyme, bay leaf and salt and pepper. Bring to a boil, then reduce the heat to medium-low, cover and simmer for 20 minutes. Discard the bay leaf.

Makes about 4 cups
Per cup: 231 calories, 4 grams fat, 8.7 grams dietary fiber

BLACK BEAN AND DRIED FRUIT SALSA

Allen Susser, chef/owner of Miami Beach's trendy Chef Allen's, came up with this low-fat gem of a side dish. Actually more than a salsa, it's a bean dish with a tropical fruit twist. If you're following the weight-loss menu, serve part of the recipe for dinner with the fish on Day 7, then have part of what's left the next day for lunch. (Freeze the rest, if you like).

Chef Allen uses dried mangoes, papayas and pineapple in the salsa. If you can't find all of them at the store, just use more of the fruit you do have. You can control the spiciness of this recipe according to your choice of chili pepper. When handling hot peppers, it's best to wear rubber gloves so you don't expose your fingers to the stinging compound that gives them their fire power. And be extra careful not to touch your eyes or lips before thoroughly washing the gloves.

6	cups water	1	tablespoon each diced dried mangoes, papayas and pineapple
¾	cup dried black beans, soaked overnight, drained		
1	bay leaf	2	teaspoons chopped fresh cilantro (coriander) or parsley (preferably flat-leaf)
¼	teaspoon dried thyme		
¼	teaspoon salt	1½	teaspoons lime juice
¾	sweet red pepper, diced	1	teaspoon ground cumin
⅓	mild or hot chili pepper (such as Anaheim or jalapeño), seeded and diced	¼	teaspoon chopped garlic

In a 3-quart saucepan, combine the water, beans, bay leaf, thyme and salt. Bring to a boil, then simmer over medium heat for 1 hour, or until the beans are tender but not soft. Drain and rinse with cold water. Discard the bay leaf.

Transfer to a large bowl. Add the red peppers, chili peppers, mangoes, papayas, pineapple, cilantro or parsley, lime juice, cumin and garlic. Refrigerate at least 30 minutes before serving.

Makes about 3 cups
Per ½ cup: 94 calories, <1 gram fat, 3.1 grams dietary fiber

THREE-BEAN SALAD

You may use any combination of beans you'd like—or even just one kind. Look for this salad on Days 7, 10 and 16 of the weight-loss menus.

¼	cup cooked chick-peas	2	scallions, chopped
¼	cup cooked kidney beans	1	teaspoon lemon juice
¼	cup cooked lima beans or ½ cup steamed green beans	1	teaspoon red-wine vinegar or balsamic vinegar
3	tablespoons chopped fresh parsley or cilantro (coriander)	1	teaspoon olive or canola oil
			Salt and pepper (to taste)

In a medium bowl, combine the chick-peas, kidney beans, lima beans or green beans, parsley or cilantro, scallions, lemon juice, vinegar, oil and salt and pepper. Let stand 15 minutes so the flavors meld.

Makes about 1 cup
Per cup: 150 calories, 5 grams fat, 6.5 grams dietary fiber

Chicken Dishes

We generally consider 3 ounces of cooked chicken to be an individual serving. When you're buying boneless, skinless breasts, you can figure that 3½ ounces of raw chicken will yield 3 ounces cooked. If you're purchasing bone-in breasts, calculate that approximately 4¼ ounces will give you 3 ounces cooked. A kitchen scale will help you figure portions fairly accurately, but if you don't have one, just read the store label and do a little arithmetic.

There are several chicken dishes in the weight-loss plan, so don't hesitate to buy more than a single serving of chicken at a time. Just individually wrap and freeze the extra pieces for upcoming meals.

GRILLED MUSTARD-LEMON CHICKEN BREAST

This is one of the easiest meals you'll ever make. If you're on the weight-loss plan, you'll find this dish on Day 4.

1½ teaspoons Dijon mustard	3½ ounces boneless, skinless chicken breast
½ teaspoon olive oil	
Salt and pepper (to taste)	

Preheat the broiler.

In a small bowl, combine the mustard, oil and salt and pepper. Add the chicken and coat both sides with the mixture. Broil about 4" from the heat for 2 minutes per side, or until the chicken is white all the way through.

Makes 1 serving
Per recipe: 169 calories, 5 grams fat, 0 grams dietary fiber

GRILLED CHICKEN STRIPS

This dish is even easier than the Grilled Mustard-Lemon Chicken Breast above. These strips are purposely plain and simple so as not to compete with the lively tropical salsa that accompanies them on Day 10. (Check your calorie level for the number of ounces of chicken on your plan.) Serve the chicken on a bed of greens.

| 3–4 | ounces boneless, skinless chicken breast, cut into 1½" strips | ½ | teaspoon olive oil |
| | | | Salt and pepper (to taste) |

Preheat the broiler.

Brush the chicken strips with the oil and season them with the salt and pepper. Broil about 4" from the heat for about 1½ minutes on each side, or until the chicken is white all the way through.

Makes 1 serving
Per serving: 160 calories, 5 grams fat, 0 grams dietary fiber

ORIENTAL CHICKEN STIR-FRY

This makes one serving for those on 1,200 or 1,500 calories. If you're on the 1,700-calorie plan, start with about 3½ ounces of chicken. Use whatever vegetables—fresh or frozen—you want. Broccoli, cauliflower, carrots, snow peas and asparagus are good choices. For even cooking, cut them into equal-size pieces.

¼	cup defatted chicken stock	2½	ounces boneless, skinless chicken breast, cut into 1½" strips
1	tablespoon soy sauce (preferably low-sodium)		
1	teaspoon honey	½	teaspoon minced garlic
½	teaspoon sesame oil	2–3	cups cut-up mixed vegetables
1	teaspoon canola oil		

In a cup, mix the stock, soy sauce, honey and sesame oil; set aside.

In a wok or medium frying pan over medium-high heat, heat the canola oil. Add the chicken and stir-fry for 2 to 3 minutes, or until white all the way through. Remove the chicken with a slotted spoon.

Add the vegetables and garlic and stir-fry for 3 minutes.

Reduce the heat to medium. Add the chicken and the stock mixture. Cover and simmer for 5 to 7 minutes, or until the vegetables are crisp-tender.

Variation: *You can easily convert this to a vegetarian dish by substituting 4 ounces of tofu for the chicken. Because the tofu is a little higher in fat, subtract 1 fat serving somewhere else on your menu for that day or the next.*

Makes about 3½ cups
Per 3½ cups: 285 calories, 10 grams fat, 6.9 grams dietary fiber

Grains

If the only grain you ever cook is white rice, you're in for a treat. There's a wide world of whole grains for you to choose from, and they'll add a new dimension to your meals. For starters, switch from white rice to brown. And don't stop with plain brown rice—try the fragrant aromatics like basmati or the colorful ones like Wehani and black japonica. Then acquaint yourself with barley, millet, whole wheat couscous, bulgur and kasha, to name a few. We think you'll really enjoy these fiber-rich gems. A general rule of thumb for cooking grains: Using twice as much water as grain, bring grain, water and salt (to taste) to a boil. Reduce heat, cover and simmer 40 minutes for whole grains, 25 minutes for processed grains.

LENTIL-BARLEY PILAF

This makes several servings, so feel free to freeze the extras. This recipe is easy enough to make, but if you'd like a super-quick dinner, try Near East's Lentil/Rice Pilaf (page 245).

6	cups water	2	bay leaves
1	cup lentils	1	teaspoon salt
¾	cup hulled barley	1–3	tablespoons minced scallions
1	whole onion, peeled		

In a 3-quart saucepan, combine the water, lentils, barley, onion, bay leaves and salt. Bring to a boil, then cover and simmer over medium-low heat for 1 hour, or until the barley is tender and the water has been absorbed.

Remove and discard the onion and bay leaves.

Fluff with a fork and serve topped with scallions.

Variation: *You may substitute brown rice for the barley. Simmer the lentils and seasonings for 15 minutes, then add the rice and cook for 45 minutes.*

Makes 5½ cups
Per cup: 221 calories, <1 gram fat, 6.6 grams dietary fiber

Bran Cocktail Brown Rice

This recipe is really easy to double or triple, so you'll have leftovers for other meals. Cooked rice keeps in the refrigerator for several days and can also be frozen, so it's worth making extra.

1	cup plus 3 tablespoons water	1	tablespoon Bran Cocktail (page 31)
⅓	cup brown rice (regular or basmati)		Pinch of salt

In a 1-quart saucepan, combine the water, rice, Bran Cocktail and salt. Bring to a boil over medium heat. Reduce the heat to low, cover with a tight-fitting lid and simmer for 40 minutes, or until the rice is tender and all the water has been absorbed. Fluff with a fork, cover and let stand for 5 minutes before serving.

Makes 1 cup
Per cup: 233 calories, 1 gram fat, 5.2 grams dietary fiber

Tomato Rice

This delicious dish is similar to Spanish rice. Look for it in the Cook's Plan on Day 8.

½	teaspoon oil		Salt and pepper (to taste)
¼	cup chopped onions	1	cup water
½	teaspoon minced garlic	⅔	cup diced tomatoes (canned low-sodium or very ripe fresh)
⅓	cup brown rice		
	Pinch of dried oregano		

In a 2-quart saucepan over medium-high heat, heat the oil. Add the onions and stir for 2 to 3 minutes, until they wilt and start to turn golden. Add the garlic and stir for 30 seconds.

Add the rice, oregano and salt and pepper; stir for 30 seconds. Stir in the water and tomatoes. Bring to a boil, then reduce the heat to medium-low, cover and simmer for 40 minutes, or until the rice is tender and all the liquid has been absorbed.

Makes 1⅓ cups
Per ½ cup: 95 calories, 3 grams fat, 2 grams dietary fiber

Homemade Muffins

As we've said elsewhere in the book, muffins are an ideal vehicle for the Bran Cocktail. With the following recipe, you can be sure of getting adequate fiber in your diet.

BRAN COCKTAIL MUFFINS

Like most other muffins, these freeze beautifully, so it's worth your while to make a whole batch. Just let them cool, then pack them in a well-sealed plastic bag. To reheat, put as many as needed in a toaster oven set at 350° for 5 to 8 minutes.

1½	cups oat bran	1¼	cups buttermilk
1	cup whole wheat flour	¼	cup water
½	cup Bran Cocktail (page 31)	¼	cup brown sugar
2	teaspoons baking soda	2–3	tablespoons mashed ripe banana
½	teaspoon salt	2	tablespoons oil
1	egg	1	cup raisins

Preheat the oven to 425°. Coat 12 muffin cups with no-stick spray or vegetable oil.

In a large bowl, combine the oat bran, flour, Bran Cocktail, baking soda and salt. Set aside.

In a small bowl, whisk together the egg, buttermilk, water, brown sugar, banana and oil. Pour over the dry ingredients and mix just until blended. Stir in the raisins.

Spoon the batter into the muffin cups, filling them ⅔ full. Bake for 12 minutes, or until the muffins have just pulled away from the sides of the pan.

Variations: *An easy way to vary this recipe is to replace the raisins with chopped dates, prunes or figs. You can also substitute applesauce for the bananas.*

Makes 12
Per muffin: 151 calories, 4 grams fat, 4 grams dietary fiber

Italian Foods

Pasta and pizza are longtime Italian favorites. Both, believe it or not, warrant a place in the weight-loss diet.

Long considered fattening, pasta is actually quite low in fat. And whole wheat pasta has lots of fiber—much more than white. For some common brands, see Appendix B on page 205. (There are many more, including quite a few imported brands. If you have trouble finding whole wheat pasta, ask your grocer to order some for you.)

You might be surprised to see pizza in this book because, generally, it *is* high in fat. But if you use low-fat cheese (a type containing less than 3 grams of fat per ounce), lots of vegetables and a whole grain crust, you have a healthy meal you can enjoy once a week.

PASTA WITH SUN-DRIED TOMATOES AND CAULIFLOWER

Sun-dried tomatoes are now easier to find—many supermarkets carry them. Buy brittle ones and soften them in boiling water for 2 minutes. If you get them packed in oil, drain well and use a bit less oil in your recipes.

1	cup rigatoni or other short, tubular pasta (preferably whole wheat)	5	sun-dried tomato halves, coarsely chopped
1	teaspoon olive oil	2	tablespoons water
1½–2	cups cauliflower florets	2	teaspoons lemon juice
½	teaspoon dried rosemary	1	tablespoon grated Parmesan cheese
1–2	scallions, finely chopped		Salt and pepper (to taste)
½	clove garlic, minced		

Cook the pasta in boiling water until just tender. Drain and set aside.

Meanwhile, heat the oil in a medium frying pan or wok over medium-high heat. Add the cauliflower and rosemary; stir constantly for 30 seconds. Add the scallions and garlic; toss gently for 1 minute.

Stir in the tomatoes and water. Reduce the heat to medium, cover and simmer for 4 minutes, or until the cauliflower is tender. Sprinkle with the lemon juice. Stir in the pasta, Parmesan and salt and pepper.

Makes 3½ cups
Per 3½ cups: 403 calories, 9 grams fat, 11.6 grams dietary fiber

AGOSTINO'S PASTA WITH BRUSSELS SPROUTS ___

Although this recipe's inventor is from Sienna, you probably won't find this dish anywhere in Italy. That's because the goat cheese it contains is a French touch, and Agostino created this recipe when he moved to Paris. A word of caution: Most goat cheese is lower in fat than regular cheese, but you'll want to check labels to make sure.

This recipe also contains brussels sprouts. And before you turn up your nose, be aware that even people who said they detested those little cabbages loved this dish.

10	ounces frozen brussels sprouts (or about 9 fresh sprouts, trimmed)	1	teaspoon olive oil
		1	clove garlic, crushed
1	cup rigatoni or other short, tubular pasta (preferably whole wheat)		Pinch of red-pepper flakes (optional)
			Salt and pepper (to taste)
2	tablespoons goat cheese, preferably reduced-fat		
2	tablespoons chopped fresh basil or parsley (preferably flat-leaf)		

Bring a large pot of water to a boil. Add the brussels sprouts and cook for 12 minutes. Add the pasta and cook for 9 minutes, or until just tender. Drain, reserving ¼ cup of the water.

Pick out the brussels sprouts and return them to the pot (off heat). Stir in the cheese, basil or parsley, oil, garlic, red-pepper flakes and salt and pepper. With a heavy fork or wooden spoon, mash most of the brussels sprouts against the sides of the pot. Add the pasta and stir well.

Stir in the reserved cooking liquid 1 tablespoon at a time until the dish has a moist consistency. Serve immediately.

Makes 1 serving
Per serving: 387 calories, 8 grams fat, 16 grams dietary fiber

GOAT-CHEESE PITA PIZZA

This pizza is very low in calories and fat. And it's a good way to use up the leftover goat cheese from Agostino's Pasta with Brussels Sprouts. Another plus: You don't have to make a crust.

1–2	tablespoons pizza or tomato sauce	¼	cup crumbled goat cheese, preferably reduced-fat
1	whole wheat pita	¼	cup chopped mushrooms
¾	cup chopped spinach or arugula	2	tablespoons finely chopped red onions

Spread the sauce on the pita. Top with the spinach or arugula. Sprinkle with the cheese, mushrooms and onions.

Broil for about 7 minutes, or until the pizza is very hot and the cheese melts.

Makes 1
Per pizza: 196 calories, 1 gram fat, 3.3 grams dietary fiber

BASIL-TOMATO SAUCE

On the Cook's Plan, use the amount of sauce specified on Days 5 and 14 and freeze the rest in small containers. If you serve ¼ cup sauce with 2 ounces whole wheat pasta, you'll get 233 calories, 2 grams fat and 7.7 grams dietary fiber. (With regular white pasta, the fiber is 3.7 grams.)

1	teaspoon olive oil	2	tablespoons chopped fresh basil or 2 teaspoons dried
½	cup finely chopped onions		
1–2	cloves garlic, minced		
1½	cups chopped plum tomatoes (canned low-sodium or very ripe fresh)		

In a 2-quart saucepan over medium-high heat, heat the oil. Add the onions and stir for about 3 minutes, or until the onions wilt and begin to turn golden. Add the garlic and stir for 30 seconds.

Reduce the heat to medium. Add the tomatoes, cover and simmer for 20 minutes. Stir in the basil and simmer for 5 minutes. Serve warm.

Makes 1½ cups
Per ¼ cup: 24 calories, 1 gram fat, 0.6 grams dietary fiber

Mexican Foods

Mexican dishes tend to be very high in fiber thanks to the beans that often appear in them. Serving these foods with rice—especially brown rice—increases the fiber even more.

CHICKEN FAJITA

If you're familiar with the juicy joy of a sizzling fajita, you'll be delighted at how easy it is to prepare one. You'll relish this addition to your Mexican repertoire. Look for this dish on Days 18 and 28 of the Cook's Plan menu.

3 tablespoons lime juice	⅓ green pepper, sliced into strips
1 tablespoon Worcestershire sauce	½ onion, sliced
1 tablespoon white-wine vinegar	1–2 teaspoons minced jalapeño peppers (wear rubber gloves to protect your hands)
2 teaspoons soy sauce (preferably low-sodium)	
½ teaspoon olive oil	1 small clove garlic, minced
1 boneless, skinless chicken breast (about 3½ ounces), cut into strips	1 flour or corn tortilla
	Fresh Tomato Salsa (page 189)

In a medium bowl, combine the lime juice, Worcestershire sauce, vinegar, soy sauce and oil. Add the chicken, green peppers, onions, jalapeños and garlic. Stir to coat the chicken and vegetables with marinade. Cover and refrigerate for at least 30 minutes, or up to 8 hours.

Remove the chicken pieces from the marinade and set aside.

Heat a medium frying pan, preferably cast-iron, over medium-high heat. Add the vegetables and marinade. Cook, stirring frequently, for 4 minutes. Add the chicken and cook, stirring, for 2 minutes, or until the chicken is white all the way through.

Soften the tortilla by microwaving it for 15 seconds or heating it in a dry frying pan for about 1 minute. Place the chicken, vegetables and salsa on the tortilla; roll to enclose the filling.

Makes 1 serving
Per fajita: 266 calories, 6 grams fat, 2.8 grams dietary fiber

Refried Beans

Serve these beans as a side dish or use them as filling for the Bean Burrito (below). Unlike many commercial refried beans, these contain no lard.

1	teaspoon canola oil	½	teaspoon minced garlic (optional)
½	onion, chopped		
¼	green pepper, seeded and finely chopped	1	cup cooked kidney beans
		¼–½	cup bean cooking liquid or water
½	jalapeño pepper, minced (optional); wear rubber gloves to protect your hands		Salt and pepper (to taste)

In a medium frying pan over medium-high heat, heat the oil. Add the onions, green peppers and jalapeño peppers, if desired; sauté for about 5 minutes. Add the garlic, if desired, and sauté for 30 seconds.

Add the beans and ¼ cup of the liquid. Reduce the heat and simmer, stirring often, for about 30 minutes. (If needed, add additional liquid.) Mash half of the beans with a fork or spoon to give the mixture a slightly lumpy consistency.

Makes 1½ cups

Per ½ cup: 97 calories, 2 grams fat, 4.6 grams dietary fiber

Bean Burrito

Look for this tasty burrito on Days 1 and 13 of the Cook's Plan.

1	corn or flour tortilla	⅓	cup chopped tomatoes
½	cup Refried Beans (above)		Fresh Tomato Salsa (page 189)
⅓	cup shredded lettuce		

To soften the tortilla, microwave it for 15 seconds or heat it in a dry frying pan for about 1 minute. Spread with beans. Sprinkle with lettuce and tomatoes. Top with some salsa and roll to enclose the filling.

Makes 1 serving

Per burrito: 187 calories, 3 grams fat, 5.2 grams dietary fiber

ALL-BEAN CHILI

This vegetarian chili is so flavorful that you won't miss having meat. Some of you might raise an eyebrow over the option to use butter instead of oil. But we feel that butter, especially when browned as it is here, contributes to a rich flavor normally provided by meat. The Bran Plan for Weight Loss is so low in cholesterol, fat and saturated fat that it's okay to have a little butter once in a while. If you really object to butter, however, by all means, substitute olive oil.

If you're following the Bran Plan for Weight Loss, check your calorie allotment for the exact serving size. And be aware that if you're allotted only a portion of the recipe, you can freeze the leftovers for another time.

1 tablespoon butter	Pinch of dried oregano
1 small onion, finely chopped	Salt and pepper (to taste)
1 teaspoon chili powder (or to taste)	1 can (15 ounces) kidney beans, undrained, or 2 cups cooked from dry
½ teaspoon ground cumin	2 tablespoons finely chopped fresh cilantro (coriander) or parsley (preferably flat-leaf)
1 clove garlic, minced	
½ cup diced tomatoes (canned low-sodium or very ripe fresh)	

In a medium frying pan over medium-high heat, heat the butter until it froths, then becomes slightly brown and clear. Turn the heat down to medium and add the onions, chili powder and cumin; stir for about 3 minutes. Add the garlic and stir for 30 seconds.

Add the tomatoes, oregano and salt and pepper. Stir in the beans (with either their canning liquid or the soaking water).

Bring to a boil, then turn the heat to medium-low, cover and simmer, stirring occasionally, for 20 to 30 minutes. If the chili seems dry, add some water. Serve sprinkled with the cilantro or parsley.

Makes about 2½ cups
Per 1¼ cups: 236 calories, 6 grams fat, 12.3 grams dietary fiber

Salsas

Salsas are an integral part of low-fat cooking, and they're a tasty treat. The Fresh Tomato Salsa is traditional and goes well with bean burritos, fajitas and other Mexican favorites. A Mano's Tropical Salsa is really closer to a sweet and spicy chutney.

FRESH TOMATO SALSA

This fresh salsa is best used within a day of making it.

2	ripe tomatoes, diced	2	tablespoons finely chopped fresh cilantro (coriander)
¼–1	jalapeño pepper, finely minced (wear rubber gloves to protect your hands)	1	tablespoon red-wine vinegar
2–3	tablespoons finely diced onions	½	teaspoon minced garlic

In a medium bowl, mix the tomatoes, jalapeño peppers, onions, cilantro, vinegar and garlic.

Makes 1½ cups
Per ¼ cup: 11 calories, 0 grams fat, 0.7 grams dietary fiber

A MANO'S TROPICAL SALSA

This recipe comes from Norm Van Aken, chef/owner of A Mano, one of the hottest restaurants in Miami Beach. Serve the salsa at room temperature. It's great with grilled fish or chicken.

½	papaya, diced	2	tablespoons minced red onions
½	mango, diced		
½	cup pineapple chunks	2	tablespoons chopped fresh cilantro (coriander) or mint or 2 teaspoons dried cilantro
¼	tomato, peeled, seeded and diced		
½	jalapeño or serrano chili pepper, minced (wear rubber gloves to protect your hands)	1	tablespoon red-wine vinegar

In a medium bowl, combine the papaya, mango, pineapple, tomatoes, peppers, onions, cilantro or mint and vinegar.

Makes 2 cups
Per ⅓ cup: 26 calories, 0 grams fat, 0.9 grams dietary fiber

Salad Dressings

The three distinguishing ingredients of a good basic vinaigrette are flavorful olive oil, an interesting vinegar and lemon juice. They contribute so much pizzazz to a salad that you can get away with very little actual dressing.

There are so many vinegars to choose from—including red wine, white wine, sherry, herbed and fruit-flavored—that you can vary your salads to suit whatever mood you're in. Balsamic vinegar is especially delicious, getting its pungent sweetness from a long aging process.

RASPBERRY TOPPING FOR FRUIT SALAD _____

When making fruit salads, give some thought to the health value of the fruits you choose. Oranges, grapefruits and strawberries, for instance, contain lots of vitamin C, a nutrient that can help prevent certain types of cancer. Cantaloupe, papayas and mangoes are good sources of beta-carotene, another cancer fighter. All contain plenty of fiber.

Adding a little lemon juice and orange juice to any fruit salad can improve its flavor and make it juicier. Letting the salad sit, covered, at room temperature for 20 minutes before serving brings out the fruits' natural flavors and gives them a chance to meld.

This topping accompanies the fruit salads on Days 2, 11 and 20. If you serve it over 1 cup of mixed kiwifruit and strawberries, the calorie count will be 107, with 6.3 grams dietary fiber and less than 1 gram fat. This topping is also delicious spooned over nonfat vanilla frozen yogurt.

⅓ cup fresh or frozen raspberries

1 tablespoon water

1 teaspoon seedless raspberry jam is best

Combine the raspberries, water and jam in a blender and process until smooth.

Makes ¼ cup

Per ¼ cup: 39 calories, 0 grams fat, 1.9 grams dietary fiber

Basic Vinaigrette _____

Use this recipe as a starting point for your own creativity. If you don't have fresh herbs, substitute a pinch of dried.

1	teaspoon olive oil	Salt and pepper (to taste)
1	teaspoon red-wine vinegar	
½	teaspoon lemon juice	
1	teaspoon minced fresh basil or other herbs or ⅓ teaspoon dried	

In a cup, whisk together the oil, vinegar, lemon juice, herbs and salt and pepper.

Makes 1 tablespoon
Per tablespoon: 40 calories, 5 grams fat, 0 grams dietary fiber

Honey-Mustard Vinaigrette _____

We particularly like this vinaigrette on a mixed green salad with chick-peas.

1	teaspoon olive oil	½	teaspoon Dijon mustard
1	teaspoon red-wine vinegar	½	teaspoon honey
1	teaspoon lemon juice		Salt and pepper (to taste)
1	teaspoon minced fresh basil or other herbs or ⅓ teaspoon dried		

In a cup, whisk together the oil, vinegar, lemon juice, herbs, mustard, honey and salt and pepper.

Makes about 1 tablespoon
Per tablespoon: 50 calories, 5 grams fat, 0 grams dietary fiber

TANGERINE VINAIGRETTE _____

Try this fruity vinaigrette with the fish and salsa on Day 7 of the Cook's Plan menu. Although you may use any type of honey, orange-blossom is particularly good.

2	teaspoons tangerine juice	Pinch of dried tarragon
1	teaspoon olive oil	Pinch of dried basil
½	teaspoon lime juice	Salt and pepper (to taste)
½	teaspoon honey	

In a cup, whisk together the tangerine juice, oil, lime juice, honey, tarragon, basil and salt and pepper.

Variation: *Replace the tangerine juice with orange juice.*

Makes about 1 tablespoon
Per tablespoon: 50 calories, 5 grams fat, 0 grams dietary fiber

Salads
_____

Salads are a staple on the Bran Plan for Weight Loss. That's because they're high in fiber, infinitely variable and certainly never boring. Whether you're making a main course, a side dish or a dessert salad, remember that the following recipes are only suggestions. You should feel free to vary the fruits and vegetables according to your own taste and what's in season. But stick to our serving size on the dressings—otherwise your daily fat intake could shoot way up.

SALMON SALAD _____

Look for this dish on Day 6 of the weight-loss menu plans. If you serve the salmon salad with two slices of whole wheat bread, you'll get 246 calories, 7 grams fat and 6.2 grams dietary fiber. When buying canned salmon, look for the type that contains bones—they are a good source of calcium.

3 ounces water-packed
salmon, drained and flaked
(about ¼ cup)

1 tablespoon diced celery

1 tablespoon diced or
shredded carrots

1 tablespoon chopped fresh
parsley or ½ teaspoon dried
herb of choice

1 teaspoon lemon juice

½ teaspoon olive oil

Salt and pepper (to taste)

In a medium bowl, mix the salmon, celery, carrots, parsley, lemon juice, oil and salt and pepper.

Makes ½ cup
Per ½ cup: 125 calories, 5 grams fat, 0.5 grams dietary fiber

CARROT-CABBAGE COLESLAW

This salad is as healthy as it is beautiful. That's because carrots are packed with cancer-fighting beta-carotene, and cabbage is thought to have other cancer-protective compounds. If you're multiplying the recipe, using the shredding blade of the food processor is a real time-saver.

1 cup thinly sliced red or
green cabbage

1 medium carrot, shredded
or julienned

1 tablespoon white-wine
vinegar

1 teaspoon canola oil

¼ teaspoon caraway seeds

¼ teaspoon celery seeds

¼ teaspoon sugar

Salt and pepper (to taste)

In a medium bowl, toss together the cabbage and carrots. Mix the vinegar, oil, caraway seeds, celery seeds, sugar and salt and pepper, and add to the vegetables. Toss well.

Makes 1½ cups
Per 1½ cups: 87 calories, 5 grams fat, 3.8 grams dietary fiber

Tuna Salad

This is the real stuff, with just a little less fat. If you use regular mayonnaise, reduce the amount to 1 teaspoon. Serving the salad with two slices of whole wheat bread gives you 274 calories, 8 grams fat and 5.9 grams dietary fiber.

3 ounces water-packed tuna, drained and flaked (about ¼ cup)

2 tablespoons chopped celery

1 tablespoon reduced-fat mayonnaise

1 tablespoon chopped sweet pickles (optional)

Pinch of dry mustard

Salt and pepper (to taste)

In a medium bowl, mix together the tuna, celery, mayonnaise, pickles, if desired, mustard and salt and pepper.

Makes ½ cup

Per ½ cup: 151 calories, 6 grams fat, 0.2 grams dietary fiber

Spinach Salad

This delicious salad is easy to throw together. You may use your favorite reduced-calorie dressing (but make sure it has no more than 5 grams of fat per serving) or one of the vinaigrettes (pages 191–92).

2 cups spinach leaves

½–1 tomato, sliced

¼ red onion, thinly sliced

1 tablespoon reduced-calorie dressing

1 hard-cooked egg, halved or sliced

1 whole grain cracker, broken into crouton-size bits (optional)

Salt and pepper (to taste)

On a salad plate, combine the spinach, tomatoes and onions. Drizzle with the dressing and toss lightly. Sprinkle the eggs with salt and pepper; arrange on the salad. Top with the cracker bits.

Makes about 3 cups

Per 3 cups: 191 calories, 11 grams fat, 5.6 grams dietary fiber

TOMATO-CUCUMBER SALAD

This tart and juicy salad is fragrant with the smells and tastes of summer. Try to find a big, ripe tomato for this one.

1	large tomato, diced, or 1 cup halved cherry tomatoes	2	teaspoons chopped fresh basil (optional)
1	gherkin (pickling) cucumber or ½ regular cucumber, cubed	2	teaspoons lemon juice
		1	teaspoon olive oil
¼	cup fresh chopped parsley		Salt and pepper (to taste)
2–3	scallions, finely chopped		

In a medium bowl, toss together the tomatoes, cucumbers, parsley, scallions and basil, if desired. Drizzle with the lemon juice and oil. Sprinkle with salt and pepper. Toss well.

Makes 1½ cups
Per 1½ cups: 105 calories, 5 grams fat, 5 grams dietary fiber

MIXED GREENS SALAD

Once you expand your salad horizons beyond iceberg lettuce, it's hard to go back. Other greens have more interesting tastes and textures. And some, like arugula, kale, spinach and other dark, leafy varieties, contain cancer-fighting beta-carotene as well as vitamin C and other nutrients. Try arugula (which has a wonderful sharp, spicy flavor) or watercress (a little peppery). Romaine lettuce provides a sweet contrast to those sharper greens, and red-leaf or red-tinged oak leaf lettuces offer a smooth softness.

Greens contain few calories, so feel free to use more than is called for. Dress them with your favorite dressing (but don't exceed 5 grams of fat per serving) or one of the vinaigrettes (pages 191–92).

1½	cups mixed greens	2–3	scallions, finely chopped
2	tablespoons chopped fresh parsley		

On a salad plate, toss together the greens, parsley and scallions.

Makes 1¾ cups
Per 1¾ cups: 20 calories, <1 gram fat, 2.3 grams dietary fiber

Seafood Dishes

Most fish is low in fat, and even higher-fat fish such as salmon and bluefish contain a type of unsaturated fat that doesn't raise cholesterol. One of our favorite ways for preparing fish is to grill it. Although a regular grill works best, the oven broiler is an acceptable alternative.

Maximize the flavor of fish—and keep it deliciously moist—by marinating it first. Several of the recipes that follow use this technique. For still more flavor, baste the fish with the marinade as it cooks. (Discard any leftover marinade.)

Broil the fish a total of eight to nine minutes per inch of thickness. That means thin fillets take just two to three minutes on each side; whole fish will naturally take longer. Fish is done when it is flaky and opaque all the way through.

GRILLED SHRIMP WITH HOT AND SWEET RED PEPPERS

Consult Day 8 of the Cook's Plan menu for your allotted amount of shrimp. If you use wooden skewers, presoak them in water for at least 30 minutes to minimize burning while the kabobs cook.

6–8	large shrimp, peeled and deveined	1	teaspoon olive oil
		1	teaspoon lemon juice
½	onion, cut lengthwise into 4 wedges	½	teaspoon ground red pepper
1	sweet red pepper, cut into 1" pieces	½	teaspoon ground black pepper
1	zucchini, cut into ½" chunks		

Preheat the broiler. Position a broiler pan so its top is about 5" from the heat. Thread the shrimp onto skewers. Set aside.

Alternate the onions, peppers and zucchini on a few skewers.

In a cup, mix the oil, lemon juice, red pepper and black pepper. Brush over the kabobs. Place them on the broiler rack and cook for 6 minutes, turning frequently and basting with the remaining oil mixture. Add the shrimp skewers to the rack and cook for 2 minutes, turning and basting frequently. Serve all immediately, either on or off the skewers.

Makes 1 serving

Per serving: 216 calories, 6 grams fat, 4.5 grams dietary fiber

BROILED FISH WITH GARLIC-LEMON MARINADE

If you really like garlic, feel free to add more. This marinade is equally delicious with any fish.

1 flounder fillet (3 to 4 ounces)	1 teaspoon olive oil
	1 clove garlic, minced
Juice of 1 lemon	Salt and pepper (to taste)

Place the fish on a plate and rub with half of the lemon juice. Refrigerate for 1 hour.

In a cup, mix the remaining lemon juice with the oil, garlic and salt and pepper.

Transfer the fish to a broiler rack. Baste with the garlic mixture. Broil for 2 to 3 minutes. Carefully flip the fish, baste and broil until done, about 2 minutes.

Makes 1 serving
Per serving: 120 calories, 6 grams fat, 0 grams dietary fiber

TROPICAL GLAZED FISH

The thick marinade used to make this fish imparts a lovely glaze to grilled or broiled fish fillets or steaks. It's especially good on salmon, tuna and swordfish. The analysis below is based on 3½ ounces of swordfish.

¼ mango, chopped	1 tablespoon minced fresh cilantro (coriander) or parsley (preferably flat-leaf)
1 teaspoon lime juice	
½ clove garlic, minced	
1 tablespoon minced sweet red peppers	Salt and pepper (to taste)
	1 fish fillet or steak (3 to 4 ounces)

In a food processor or blender, puree the mango, lime juice and garlic. Transfer to a shallow bowl. Stir in the peppers, cilantro or parsley and salt and pepper. Add the fish and turn to coat both sides. Refrigerate for at least 30 minutes.

Transfer the fish to a broiler rack or grill. Baste with the marinade mixture. Cook for 2 to 3 minutes. Carefully flip the fish, baste and cook until cooked through.

Makes 1 serving
Per serving: 169 calories, 5 grams fat, 1.4 grams dietary fiber

CRAIG CLAIBORNE'S LINGUINE WITH CLAM SAUCE

Here's a recipe this famous chef created for Longevity *magazine. If you use whole wheat pasta, the fiber will increase to 5.3 grams.*

6 shucked littleneck clams (plus liquid)	2 ounces linguine*
Bottled clam juice (optional)	½ teaspoon butter, softened
½ teaspoon cornstarch	1½ teaspoons cognac (optional)
1 teaspoon olive oil	2 tablespoons chopped fresh parsley
2 teaspoons minced garlic	
⅛ teaspoon red-pepper flakes	

Drain the clams and measure the liquid. If there is less than ⅓ cup, add bottled clam juice to make up the difference. Mix in the cornstarch until well dissolved.

In a 1-quart saucepan over medium heat, heat the oil. Stir in the garlic and red-pepper flakes. Cook, stirring, for about 30 seconds. Stir in the liquid and cook, stirring constantly, until slightly thickened. Set aside.

Meanwhile, cook the linguine in boiling water until just tender, according to package directions. Drain and place in a large bowl. Add the butter and mix well.

Add the clams and cognac, if desired, to the saucepan. Stir over heat very briefly until the clams are just cooked but not toughened. Pour over the pasta and toss to mix well. Sprinkle with the parsley.

Makes 1½ cups

Per 1½ cups: 293 calories, 8 grams fat, 2.3 grams dietary fiber

Use this circle for a perfect measure of spaghetti or linguine. This works only for dry pasta, not the fresh type. Remove a bundle of pasta from the package and neatly stack it. Put one end of the bundle on this circle, adding or subtracting pasta until the bundle just fits in the cirle (and you can see the outline of the circle). If you're using angel hair, use a slightly smaller bundle.

PASTA WITH SMOKED SALMON AND WATERCRESS

Many recipes for pasta with smoked salmon contain heavy cream. We prefer this version. It's so flavorful, we guarantee you'll forget that this is a low-fat dish. Cooking time for the pasta will vary depending on whether you're using regular spaghetti or angel hair. Follow package directions to keep from overcooking the noodles.

2 ounces whole wheat spaghetti or angel hair (see previous page for tip on measuring pasta)	½ bunch watercress, coarsely chopped
1 teaspoon olive oil	2 ounces smoked salmon, cut into 1" long strips
¼ teaspoon minced garlic	Salt and pepper (to taste)

Cook the pasta in boiling water until just tender. Drain, reserving about 3 tablespoons of the water. Place the pasta in a large bowl.

Meanwhile, heat the oil in a small frying pan over medium heat. Add the garlic and stir constantly for 30 seconds. Add the watercress and stir frequently for 2 minutes, or until the watercress wilts.

Spoon over the pasta. Add the salmon and salt and pepper. Toss well. Sprinkle with 1 tablespoon of the cooking liquid. If the pasta still feels dry, add another 1 or 2 tablespoons until you like the consistency.

Makes 1 serving
Per serving: 344 calories, 8.5 grams fat, 3.9 grams dietary fiber

SHELLFISH RISOTTO

You can easily multiply this recipe. Risotto is a Northern Italian dish made of rice that is stirred constantly as it slowly absorbs liquid. Many risotto recipes are full of butter and cream, but this one is not. And although making risotto is a time-consuming process, the dish won't really take you any longer than most other meals to prepare. It's just that you'll get an extra measure of exercise during that time.

Traditional risotto recipes use Arborio rice, a short-grain variety often found in specialty stores. You may substitute regular long-grain rice (we like the parboiled type, such as Uncle Ben's). If you're buying clams in the shell, count on three large cherrystones (about 4 ounces) per serving. If the clams are already shucked, ask your fish merchant to give you some of the liquid they come in. If none is available, you can use bottled clam juice.

⅓ cup coarsely chopped shucked clams (plus liquid)	⅓ cup diced tomatoes (canned low-sodium or very ripe fresh)
Bottled clam juice (optional)	Pinch of dried oregano
1 teaspoon olive oil	¼ cup Arborio rice
2 tablespoons chopped onions	2 tablespoons chopped fresh parsley or 2 teaspoons dried
3 large sea scallops or 6 bay scallops	Salt and pepper (to taste)
¼ cup thinly sliced mushooms	
½ teaspoon finely minced garlic	

Drain the clams, reserving the liquid. Measure the liquid, and add enough water or bottled clam juice to equal 1 cup. Place the liquid in a 1-quart saucepan and bring to a simmer.

In a 2-quart saucepan over medium heat, heat the oil. Add the onions and stir for about 3 minutes. Stir in the scallops, mushrooms, garlic and the clams. Cook, stirring, for 2 minutes.

Remove the scallop/clam mixture and set aside. Add the tomatoes and oregano to the pan. Bring to a boil. Stir in the rice.

Stir in a few tablespoons of the hot clam juice. Continue to cook, stirring constantly, until the liquid has been absorbed. Repeat until all the clam juice has been used and the rice is cooked but still a little firm to the bite. This process will take 20 to 25 minutes.

Add back the scallops and clams. Season with the parsley and salt and pepper. Cook for 1 minute to heat everything. The consistency should be moist and sticky but not soupy. Turn off the heat, cover the pot and let stand for 1 to 2 minutes before serving.

Variation: *If you're not up for the exertion, just prepare a pot of regular rice. While it's cooking, sauté the onions, mushrooms and garlic until soft. Then add the tomatoes and oregano; bring to a boil. Stir in the seafood and cook for 2 minutes. Combine this mixture with the cooked rice and serve.*

Makes 2 cups
Per 2 cups: 390 calories, 7 grams fat, 1.6 grams dietary fiber

Vegetable Entrée and Side Dishes

Steamed vegetables are so easy to prepare—and so delicious—that you can enjoy them often. No matter what type you're cooking, the procedure is the same. You may choose raw or frozen vegetables. If they're not too large, keep them whole. Otherwise, cut them into uniform pieces. Use a pot that comes with a perforated steamer insert or buy a folding metal insert for your regular saucepans. Place about an inch of water in your pan (make sure it's below the level of the steamer). Add the vegetables, cover and bring to a boil. Cook, checking frequently, until the vegetables are just tender. For most vegetables that's five to seven minutes. Serve them hot with a spritz of fresh lemon juice and, if desired, a sprinkle of salt and pepper.

OLIVER'S ALTOGETHER HEALTHY STIR-FRY

This is what Dr. Alabaster's family clamors for when he's the chef. You can easily multiply the recipe. If you're following the Cook's Plan, this dish appears on Days 6 and 24. Double-check the total amount of vegetables for your particular calorie level. If you don't have fresh vegetables on hand, you may use 2½ cups of a frozen cauliflower, broccoli and carrot mixture. Serving these vegetables over brown rice will increase the calories to 351, the fat to 6 grams and the dietary fiber to 10.5 grams.

1	teaspoon canola oil	¼	teaspoon dried thyme
¼	teaspoon minced garlic		Salt and pepper (to taste)
1	cup broccoli florets		Pinch of red-pepper flakes (optional)
1	cup cauliflower florets		
½	cup chopped carrots	2	tablespoons water
¼	teaspoon cumin seeds		

In a wok or large frying pan over medium-high heat, heat the oil. Add the garlic and stir for 30 seconds. Add the broccoli, cauliflower, carrots, cumin seeds, thyme, salt and pepper and red-pepper flakes. Stir for 1 minute.

Reduce the heat to medium-low, add the water and cover loosely. Cook for 7 minutes, or until the vegetables are just tender.

Makes 2½ cups
Per 2½ cups: 119 calories, 5 grams fat, 7.2 grams dietary fiber.

Yogurt Recipes

Nonfat yogurt is indispensable for anyone on a weight-loss program. It's a perfectly acceptable substitute for high-fat sour cream. And if you drain off the excess whey (in a sieve lined with cheesecloth or a paper coffee filter), you can make yogurt cheese—which has the luscious, thick texture of cream cheese. Yogurt goes equally well with fruits and vegetables, so it's a natural for everything from snacks and desserts to main courses and side dishes. The following are some of our favorite ways to use this dairy product.

BANANA SHAKE

This calcium-packed shake makes a quick breakfast or snack.

½ cup nonfat yogurt

½ cup skim milk

½ ripe banana, sliced

4 fresh or frozen strawberries

1 tablespoon frozen orange juice concentrate

1 teaspoon honey

In a blender, combine the yogurt, milk, bananas, strawberries, orange juice concentrate and honey. Blend until smooth. To serve, pour into a tall glass.

Makes 1⅓ cups

Per 1⅓ cups: 209 calories, <1 gram fat, 1.2 grams dietary fiber

MINT-YOGURT TOPPING

Use this savory yogurt mixture in place of sour cream on baked potatoes, baked yams and other vegetables. You may also use it as a topping for pilafs and other grain dishes. As with the Yogurt Topping for Fruit (page 204), you can increase the fiber content by adding a little Bran Cocktail (page 31) to the recipe.

¼ cup nonfat yogurt

2 tablespoons finely diced cucumbers

2 teaspoons ice water

½ teaspoon dried mint

½ clove garlic, crushed (optional)

¼ teaspoon salt

In a small bowl, mix the yogurt, cucumbers, water, mint, garlic, if desired, and salt. Chill; it keeps about 2 days in the refrigerator.

Makes 7 tablespoons

Per 7 tablespoons: 33 calories, <1 gram fat, 0.1 grams dietary fiber

YOGURT-DILL TOPPING

Use this mixture in the same ways as the Mint-Yogurt Topping (page 203).

¼ cup nonfat yogurt   Salt (to taste)

1 teaspoon chopped fresh
  dill or ½ teaspoon dried

In a cup, mix the yogurt, dill and salt. Chill.

Makes ¼ cup
Per ¼ cup: 31 calories, <1 gram fat, 0 grams dietary fiber

YOGURT TOPPING FOR FRUIT

This simple topping is a snap to throw together. The recipe makes enough for 1 cup of fruit—use whatever's in season. For an extra amount of fiber, stir some Bran Cocktail (page 31) into the topping.

¼ cup nonfat yogurt   ¼ teaspoon vanilla

1 teaspoon honey

In a cup, mix the yogurt, honey and vanilla. Spoon over fruit.

Variation: *You could replace the strawberries accompanying this sauce in the Cook's Plan with other fruit, such as raspberries, peach slices or pineapple chunks.*

Makes ¼ cup
Per ¼ cup: 53 calories, <1 gram fat, 0 grams dietary fiber

B

Guide to Low-Fat, High-Fiber Brand-Name Foods

Here's where you'll find foods to use in the Bran Plan for Weight Weight Loss in chapter 6 and the 28 Days of Weight-Loss Menus in chapter 7. If you're following the Take-Out Plan, which minimizes cooking and relies on frozen dinners and canned foods, you'll find the appropriate prepared foods here. The Cook's Plan (chapter 7) also occasionally calls for foods listed here. If you can't find the brand-names, use the general calorie and fat guidelines to find a good substitute.

For instance, breakfast on Day 1 of both the Take-Out and Cook's Plans calls for bran cereal and refers you here. Checking "Cereals," you can see that we've listed only high-fiber cereals. You may choose any of the cereals listed, or another cereal that fits the fat and fiber guidelines given in those sections. The same applies for all the other foods.

The brand-name foods listed here represent the kind of reduced-fat, higher-fiber choices now available, but the lists are not comprehensive. Plus, the same brand may have higher-fat and -calorie items, so read labels carefully. Manufacturers are constantly reformulating products—don't be surprised if calorie and fat values change.

Beans and Legumes

Food	Serving	Calories	Total Fat (g)	Saturated Fat (g)	Fiber (g)
Plain Canned Beans					
Progresso					
Black	½ cup	90	1	<1	6.5
Cannellini (white kidney)	½ cup	80	<1	<1	6.5
Fava	½ cup	90	<1	<1	12.0
Red kidney	½ cup	100	<1	<1	7.0
Prepared Canned Beans					
Hanover					
Baked Barbecue Beans	½ cup	160	2	—	5.2
Baked Beans with Brown Sugar and Bacon	½ cup	140	1	—	6.0
Baked Vegetarian Beans	½ cup	130	0	0	5.7
Pork and Beans	½ cup	120	1	—	6.0
Health Valley					
Fat-Free Boston Baked Beans with Honey	7.5 oz.	190	<1	—	5.0
Fat-Free Fast Menu, Hearty Lentils and Garden Vegetables	7.5 oz.	150	3	—	15.5
Fat-Free Fast Menu, Western Black Beans with Vegetables	7.5 oz.	150	3	—	14.5

Food	Serving (oz.)	Calories	Total Fat (g)	Saturated Fat (g)	Fiber (g)
Tofu Fast Meals, Baked Beans with Tofu Weiners	7.5 oz.	140	3	—	15.8
Heinz					
Vegetarian Beans	½ cup	120	2	—	5.1
Van Camp's					
New Orleans-Style Red Kidney Beans	½ cup	90	<1	—	—
Pork and Beans	½ cup	110	<1	—	6.0

NOTE: A dash indicates that no data are available for that food component.

Beef, Pork and Veal

Food	Serving (oz.)	Calories	Total Fat (g)	Saturated Fat (g)	Fiber (g)
Beef					
Lean Cuts					
Eye round	3.0	150	5.0	2.0	0
Round tip	3.0	155	5.5	2.0	0
Shank cross cut	3.0	170	5.5	2.0	0
Top round	3.0	175	5.0	1.5	0

(continued)

Beef, Pork and Veal—Continued

Food	Serving	Calories	Total Fat (g)	Saturated Fat (g)	Fiber (g)
Beef—Continued					
Frozen Entrées					
Budget Gourmet					
Beef Cantonese	9.0	270	9.0	—	—
Budget Gourmet Light and Healthy					
Sirloin Salisbury Steak	11.0	280	9.0	4.0	0
Oriental Beef	10.0	290	8.0	3.0	—
Eating Right					
Beef Sirloin Tips over Noodles	9.0	280	9.0	3.0	—
Healthy Choice					
Beef Enchilada	12.75	350	5.0	—	—
Beef Fajita	7.0	210	9.0	—	—
Lean Cuisine					
Oriental Beef with Vegetables and Rice	8.6	290	9.0	2.0	—

	Serving	Calories	Total Fat (g)	Saturated Fat (g)	Fiber (g)
Pork					
Ham, smoked	3.0	135	4.5	1.5	0
Tenderloin	3.0	140	4.0	1.5	0
Veal					
Arm chop	3.0	140	5.0	2.0	0
Cutlet	3.0	130	3.0	1.0	0

NOTES: All values are for cooked meats. A dash indicates that no data are available for that food component.

Breads, English Muffins and Rolls

Food	Serving	Calories	Total Fat (g)	Saturated Fat (g)	Fiber (g)
Breads					
Rye and Pumpernickel					
Pepperidge Farm					
Family Rye, Seedless Rye	2 slices (2.3 oz.)	160	2	—	4.0
Rubschlager					
Westphalian Pumpernickel	2 slices (2 oz.)	140	2	0	6.0

(continued)

Breads, English Muffins and Rolls—Continued

Food	Serving	Calories	Total Fat (g)	Saturated Fat (g)	Fiber (g)
Breads—Continued					
Wheat, Whole Wheat and Multigrain					
Arnold's					
Bran'nola Nutty Grains	2 slices (2.6 oz.)	160	3	<1	6.0
Honey Wheat Berry	2 slices (2.3 oz.)	160	2	<1	5.0
Light Golden Wheat, Oatmeal Light	2 slices (1.5 oz.)	80	1	<1	4.0
Stoneground 100% Whole Wheat	2 slices (1.5 oz.)	100	1	<1	3.0
Blue Ribbon					
Lite Wheat	2 slices (1.5 oz.)	80	1	—	6.5
B & M					
Brown Bread, Raisin	1 slice (1.6 oz.)	80	0	0	2.0

	Serving	Calories			
Less					
Reduced-Calorie Oat Bran	2 slices (1.6 oz.)	80	1	—	4.0
Old Tyme					
Split Top Wheat	2 slices (1.8 oz.)	140	2	—	2.0
Pepperidge Farm					
100% Whole Wheat	2 slices (1.8 oz.)	120	2	—	4.0
Wheat (32 oz. loaf)	2 slices (1.8 oz.)	140	2	—	4.0
Roman Meal					
Light Wheat	2 slices (1.6 oz.)	80	<1	<1	5.5
English Muffins					
Arnold's					
Bran'nola	1 (2.3 oz.)	160	1	—	2.0

(continued)

Breads, English Muffins and Rolls—Continued

Food	Serving	Calories	Total Fat (g)	Saturated Fat (g)	Fiber (g)
English Muffins—Continued					
Thomas'					
Honey Wheat	1 (2 oz.)	120	1	<1	2.5
Oat Bran	1 (2 oz.)	120	1	<1	3.0
Pumpernickel	1 (2 oz.)	120	<1	<1	3.0
Pita					
Thomas'					
Sahara Whole Wheat Pita (mini loaves)	2 (2 oz.)	130	1	<1	5.0
Rolls					
Arnold's					
Bran'nola Hot Dog	1 (1.6 oz.)	100	1	<1	3.0
Bran'nola with Bran	1 (1.6 oz.)	100	<1	<1	3.0

NOTE: A dash indicates that no data are available for that food component.

Cereals

Food	Serving	Calories	Total Fat (g)	Saturated Fat (g)	Fiber (g)
Ready-to-Eat Cereals					
Very High Fiber (9 g and over)					
Kellogg's					
All-Bran	⅓ cup (1 oz.)	70	1	0	9.0
All-Bran with Extra Fiber	½ cup (1 oz.)	50	0	0	14.0
Bran Buds	⅓ cup (1 oz.)	70	1	0	11.0
General Mills					
Fiber One	½ cup (1 oz.)	60	1	—	13.0
Health Valley					
Fruit & Fitness Cereal	¾ cup (2 oz.)	220	4	—	10.8
Nabisco					
100% Bran	⅓ cup (1 oz.)	70	1	0	10.0

(continued)

Cereals—Continued

Food	Serving	Calories	Total Fat (g)	Saturated Fat (g)	Fiber (g)
Ready-to-Eat Cereals—Continued					
High Fiber (3 to 8 g)					
Kellogg's					
Apple Raisin Crisp	⅔ cup (1.3 oz.)	130	0	0	3.0
Blueberry Squares	½ cup (1 oz.)	90	0	0	3.0
Bran Flakes	⅔ cup (1 oz.)	90	0	0	5.0
Common Sense Oat Bran	¾ cup (1.3 oz.)	100	1	0	3.0
Common Sense Oat Bran with Raisins	¾ cup (1.3 oz.)	130	1	0	3.0
Fiberwise	⅔ cup (1 oz.)	90	1	0	5.0
Fruitful Bran	⅔ cup (1 oz.)	120	1	—	5.0

		Calories			
Mueslix Crispy Blend	2/3 cup (1.5 oz.)	160	2	0	3.0
Mueslix Golden Crunch	1/2 cup (1.2 oz.)	120	2	0	3.0
Nutri-Grain Almond Raisin	2/3 cup (1.4 oz.)	140	2	0	3.0
Nutri-Grain Raisin Bran	2/3 cup (1.4 oz.)	130	1	0	5.0
Nutri-Grain Wheat	2/3 cup (1 oz.)	90	0	0	3.0
Raisin Bran	3/4 cup (1.4 oz.)	120	1	0	5.0
Whole Grain Shredded Wheat	1/2 cup (1 oz.)	90	0	0	4.0
Barbara's					
Shredded Wheat	2 biscuits (1.4 oz.)	140	1	0	5.0
General Mills					
Total (wheat)	1 cup (1 oz.)	100	1	—	3.0
Total Raisin Bran	1 cup (1.5 oz.)	140	1	—	4.0
Wheaties	1 cup (1 oz.)	100	1	—	3.0

(continued)

Cereals—Continued

Food	Serving	Calories	Total Fat (g)	Saturated Fat (g)	Fiber (g)
Ready-to-Eat Cereals—Continued					
High Fiber (3 to 8 g)—Continued					
Health Valley					
Amaranth Cereal with Bananas	¼ cup (1 oz.)	110	2	—	4.2
Fat-Free 10 Bran Cereal, Regular	½ cup (1 oz.)	90	<1	—	5.0
Healthy O's Children's Cereal	½ cup (1 oz.)	90	1	—	3.4
No-Fat-Added Healthy Crunch (Almond Date, Apple Cinnamon)	¼ cup (1 oz.)	90	1	—	3.5
No-Fat-Added Orangeola, Almonds and Dates	¼ cup (1 oz.)	90	1	—	3.0
No-Fat-Added Real Oat Bran, Almond Flavor Crunch	¼ cup (1 oz.)	90	1	—	3.0
No-Fat-Added Real Oat Bran, Hawaiian Fruit	¼ cup (1 oz.)	100	1	—	4.0
No-Fat-Added Real Oat Bran, Raisin	¼ cup (1.2 oz.)	100	1	—	4.0

No-Fat-Added Swiss Breakfast, Raisin	¼ cup (1 oz.)	80	1	—	3.0
Oat Bran Flakes with Almonds and Dates	¾ cup (1 oz.)	90	1	—	3.7
100% Natural Bran Cereal with Apples and Cinnamon	¼ cup (1 oz.)	90	1	—	5.1
100% Organic Bran Cereal with Raisins	¼ cup (1 oz.)	90	<1	—	5.1
100% Organic Corn Flakes	¾ cup (1 oz.)	90	<1	—	4.0
100% Organic Fiber 7 Flakes (with or without raisins)	¾ cup (1 oz.)	90	<1	—	5.0
100% Organic Oat Bran Flakes (with or without raisins)	¾ cup (1 oz.)	90	<1	—	3.7
100% Organic Oat Bran O's, Regular	½ cup (1 oz.)	90	<1	—	3.7
Nabisco					
Fruit Wheats (Blueberry, Raspberry)	½ cup (1 oz.)	90	0	0	3.0
Shredded Wheat	1 biscuit (.8 oz.)	80	1	—	3.0
Shredded Wheat 'N Bran	⅔ cup (1 oz.)	90	0	0	4.0
Spoon Size Shredded Wheat	⅔ cup (1 oz.)	90	1	0	3.0

(continued)

Cereals—Continued

Food	Serving	Calories	Total Fat (g)	Saturated Fat (g)	Fiber (g)
Ready-to-Eat Cereals—Continued					
High Fiber (3 to 8 g)—Continued					
Post					
Fruit & Fibre (Dates, Raisins and Walnuts; Peaches, Raisins and Almonds)	⅔ cup (1.2 oz.)	120	2	—	4.5
Grape-Nuts	¼ cup (1 oz.)	110	0	—	3.0
Ralston					
Multi-Bran Chex	⅔ cup (1 oz.)	90	0	0	4.0
Hot Cereals					
Multigrain					
Arrowhead Mills					
4-Grain Cereal	½ cup (¼ cup dry)	94	1	0	7.4
7-Grain Cereal	½ cup (¼ cup dry)	100	1	0	4.0

Food	Serving Size	Calories			
Oat Bran					
Arrowhead Mills	¾ cup (⅓ cup dry)	110	1	0	7.9
Mother's	⅔ cup (⅓ cup dry)	90	2	<1	4.0
Quaker					
Instant	⅔ cup (⅓ cup dry)	100	2	<1	3.5
Raisin Cinnamon	1 packet (1.23 oz.)	120	2	—	3.5
3-Minute Brand	⅔ cup (⅓ cup dry)	90	2	—	4.0
Oatmeal, Instant					
Arrowhead Mills					
Apple Spice	¾ cup (⅓ cup dry)	130	2	0	3.4
Cinnamon Raisin and Almond	¾ cup (⅓ cup dry)	140	3	0	4.3
Regular	¾ cup (⅓ cup dry)	100	2	0	4.3

(continued)

Cereals—Continued

Food	Serving	Calories	Total Fat (g)	Saturated Fat (g)	Fiber (g)
Hot Cereals—Continued					
Oatmeal, Instant—Continued					
Quaker					
Apple Cinnamon	⅔ cup (1 packet)	120	2	<1	3.0
Peaches and Cream	⅔ cup (1 packet)	130	2	<1	2.5
Raisin Spice	⅔ cup (1 packet)	150	2	<1	3.0
Oatmeal, Quick					
Quaker					
Quick Oats	⅔ cup (⅓ cup dry)	100	2	<1	2.5
Wheat					
Wheatena	¼ cup (1 oz. dry)	100	1	0	4.0

NOTE: A dash indicates that no data are available for that food component.

Cheese

Food	Serving (oz.)	Calories	Total Fat (g)	Saturated Fat (g)	Fiber (g)
Waxy or Hard Cheese					
Laughing Cow					
Reduced-Calorie Wedge	1	40	3	2	0
Polly-O					
Fat-free Mozzarella	1	40	0	—	0
Sapsago	1	41	0	—	0
Soft and Moist Cheese					
Friendship					
Farmer's cheese	1	40	3	—	0
Fromage blanc	1	19	0	—	0
Maggio					
Part-Skim Ricotta	1	40	3	—	0
Polly-O					
Fat-Free Ricotta	1	25	0	—	0

(continued)

Cheese—Continued

Food	Serving (oz.)	Calories	Total Fat (g)	Saturated Fat (g)	Fiber (g)
Goat Cheese					
Coach Farm Reduced-Fat	1	34	1	—	0
Low-Fat Cottage Cheese					
Friendship					
Large-Curd Pot Style	4	100	2	—	0
Light n'Lively					
1% Milkfat	4	80	2	1	0
Nonfat	4	90	0	0	0

NOTE: A dash indicates that no data are available for that food component.

Chicken and Turkey

Food	Serving (oz.)	Calories	Total Fat (g)	Saturated Fat (g)	Fiber (g)
Chicken					
Fresh, Skinless*					
White meat	3.0	145	4.0	—	0
Dark meat	3.0	175	8.5	—	0

Frozen Entrées				
Birds Eye				
Chicken Teriyaki	7.0	160	4.0	1	4
Budget Gourmet				
Teriyaki Chicken	11.0	270	6.0	—	—
Budget Gourmet Light and Healthy				
Chicken Breast Fettucini	11.0	240	7.0	3	—
Chicken Breast Parmesan	11.0	260	8.0	3	—
Teriyaki Chicken	11.0	300	8.0	1	—
Mandarin Chicken	10.0	240	5.0	1	—
Eating Right				
Chicken Breast with Vegetables	9.0	200	4.0	1	—
Healthy Balance				
Chicken Mesquite	10.0	260	5.0	—	—
Sweet/Sour Chicken	10.0	260	6.0	—	—
Healthy Choice				
Chicken Dijon	11.0	250	3.0	1	—
Chicken Fajita	7.0	200	3.0	—	—
Chicken à l'Orange	9.0	240	2.0	1	—
Chicken Parmigiana	11.5	270	6.0	—	—

(continued)

Chicken and Turkey—Continued

Food	Serving (oz.)	Calories	Total Fat (g)	Saturated Fat (g)	Fiber (g)
Chicken—Continued					
Frozen Entrées—Continued					
Chicken and Pasta Divan	11.5	310	4.0	2	—
Chicken and Vegetables	11.5	210	1.0	—	—
Glazed Chicken	8.5	220	3.0	1	—
Herb-Roasted Chicken	12.3	290	4.0	—	—
Mandarin Chicken	11.0	260	2.0	—	—
Oriental Chicken	11.25	230	1.0	—	—
Lean Cuisine					
Chicken in Barbecue Sauce	8.75	260	6.0	1	—
Chicken Chow Mein with Rice	9.0	240	5.0	1	—
Chicken Enchiladas	9.9	290	9.0	3	—
Chicken à l'Orange with Almond Rice	8.0	280	4.0	1	—
Chicken Tenderloins in Herb Cream Sauce	9.5	260	5.0	2	—
Chicken and Vegetables with Vermicelli	11.8	250	6.0	3	—
Fiesta Chicken	8.5	240	5.0	2	—
Glazed Chicken with Vegetable Rice	8.5	260	8.0	2	—

Turkey					
Fresh, skinless*					
White meat	3.0	135	2.5	—	0
Dark meat	3.0	160	6.0	—	0
Ground, breast (7% to 8% fat by weight)	3.0	150	6.0	—	0
Frozen Entrées					
Budget Gourmet Light and Healthy					
Stuffed Turkey Breast	11.0	230	6.0	2	—
Budget Gourmet Slim Selects					
Glazed Turkey	9.0	270	5.0	—	—
Healthy Choice					
Breast of Turkey	10.5	290	5.0	2	—
Fettucine with Turkey and Vegetables Pasta Classic	12.5	240	6.0	—	—

*All values are for cooked meats.

NOTE: A dash indicates that no data are available for that food component.

(continued)

Cold Cuts and Deli Meats

Food	Serving	Calories	Total Fat (g)	Saturated Fat (g)	Fiber (g)
Chicken					
Louis Rich Thin Sliced					
Chicken Breast	3 slices (1 oz.)	25	<1	<1	—
Original Chicken Breast	2 slices (0.8 oz.)	25	<1	<1	—
Rich's					
Deluxe Chicken Breast	1 slice (1 oz.)	30	<1	<1	0
Ham					
DAK					
Slender Slice Ham	1 oz.	30	<1	<1	—
Sliced Imported Ham	1 oz.	25	<1	<1	0
Oscar Mayer					
Thin Sliced Boiled or Smoked Ham	2 slices (0.8 oz.)	25	<1	<1	—

Turkey
Hillshire Farm

Smoked Turkey Breast	1 slice (1 oz.)	30	1	<1	—

Louis Rich

Oven Roasted Turkey Breast	1 slice (1 oz.)	30	<1	<1	0
Smoked Turkey Breast, Turkey Ham	1 slice (1 oz.)	35	1	<1	0

Louis Rich Thin Sliced

Original Turkey Breast	2 slices (0.8 oz.)	25	<1	<1	—
Smoked Turkey Breast	2 slices (0.8 oz.)	20	<1	<1	—
Turkey Ham	2 slices (0.7 oz.)	25	<1	<1	0

Mr. Turkey

Oven-Roast Turkey Breast	3 slices (1 oz.)	30	<1	<1	0
Smoked Turkey Ham	1 oz.	30	<1	<1	0
Turkey Breast (Smoked)	3 slices (1 oz.)	30	<1	<1	—

(continued)

Cold Cuts and Deli Meats—Continued

Food	Serving	Calories	Total Fat (g)	Saturated Fat (g)	Fiber (g)
Turkey—Continued					
Oscar Mayer					
Thin Sliced Turkey	2 slices (0.8 oz.)	25	<1	<1	—
Rich's					
Honey-Cured Turkey Ham	1 slice (0.7 oz.)	25	<1	<1	0
Rocco					
Turkey Breast Supreme (Service Deli)	1 oz.	25	<1	<1	0
Round Hill					
Turkey Breast, no salt added (Service Deli)	1 oz.	30	<1	<1	0

NOTE: A dash indicates that no data are available for that food component.

Crackers, Crispbreads and Corn and Rice Cakes

Food	Serving	Calories	Total Fat (g)	Saturated Fat (g)	Fiber (g)
Crackers					
Health Valley					
Fat-Free Organic Crackers (Whole-Wheat with Vegetables; Whole-Wheat with Onion, Cheese, Herb)	0.5 oz.	40	0	—	1.9
Horowitz and Margareten Matzo					
Whole Wheat	½ piece (0.5 oz.)	60	<1	<1	2.0
Ideal					
Fiber Thins	2 (0.4 oz.)	40	<1	<1	2.0
Nabisco					
Triscuit Deli Style Rye	3 (0.5 oz.)	60	2	—	2.0
Ry-Krisp					
Original	2 triple (0.5 oz.)	40	0	0	3.0
Venus					
Bran Wafers, no salt	5 (0.5 oz.)	60	<1	<1	2.0

(continued)

Crackers, Crispbreads and Corn and Rice Cakes—Continued

Food	Serving	Calories	Total Fat (g)	Saturated Fat (g)	Fiber (g)
Crispbreads					
Finn Crisps					
Dark, Dark with Caraway Seeds	2 pieces (0.4 oz.)	40	0	0	—
Wasa					
Golden Rye	1 slice (0.4 oz.)	35	0	0	1.5
Hearty Rye	1 slice (0.6 oz.)	50	0	0	2.5
Lite Rye	1 slice (0.3 oz.)	25	0	0	1.0
Royal	¼ piece	20	0	0	1.5
Corn, Rice, Wheat and Rye Cakes					
Chico-San					
Popcorn Cake, Cheddar	1 (0.4 oz.)	50	2	—	0.5
Popcorn and Rice Cake, salted	2 (0.6 oz.)	70	<1	<1	0.5

Food	Serving	Calories	Total Fat (g)	Saturated Fat (g)	Fiber (g)
Hain					
Mini Apple Cinnamon Cake, Mini Honey Nut Cake	5 (0.5 oz.)	60	<1	<1	—
Mini Popcorn Cake	5 (0.5 oz.)	60	1	—	—
Mini Teriyaki Cake	5 (0.5 oz.)	50	<1	<1	—
Mother's					
Buckwheat Rice Cake, no salt; Plain Rice Cake, no salt; Sesame Rice Cake; Sesame Rice Cake, no salt	2 (0.6 oz.)	70	<1	<1	0.5
Quaker					
Corn Cake	2 (0.6 oz.)	70	<1	<1	0.5

NOTE: A dash indicates that no data are available for that food component.

Frozen Yogurt, Fruit Ices, Ice Milk and Sorbets

Food	Serving	Calories	Total Fat (g)	Saturated Fat (g)	Fiber (g)
Frozen Yogurt					
Columbo					
Soft-serve nonfat, all flavors	½ cup	100	0	—	—
Soft-serve low-fat, all flavors	½ cup	110	2	—	—
Gourmet Wild Raspberry, Gourmet Strawberry Passion (hardpack)	½ cup	133	3	—	—

(continued)

Frozen Yogurt, Fruit Ices, Ice Milk and Sorbets—Continued

Food	Serving	Calories	Total Fat (g)	Saturated Fat (g)	Fiber (g)
Frozen Yogurt—Continued					
Elan					
Chocolate, Decaffeinated Coffee, Vanilla	½ cup	130	3	—	—
Edy's Nonfat					
Chocolate, Vanilla	½ cup	110	0	—	0
Edy's Frozen Yogurt Inspirations					
Chocolate, Strawberry, Vanilla	½ cup	110	3	—	0
Fruit Ices					
Dole Fruit'N Cream Bars					
Peach, Strawberry	1 (2.3 oz.)	90	1	—	—
Dole Fruit'N Juice Bars					
Peach-Passion, Pineapple Orange Banana, Raspberry, Strawberry	1 (2.5 oz.)	70	<1	<1	—

Ice Milk

Healthy Choice

Chocolate, Praline and Caramel	½ cup	130	2	1	—
Vanilla, Neapolitan	½ cup	120	2	1	—

Hood Free

Boston Brownie Sundae, Praline Pecan Delight	½ cup	120	1	—	—
Heavenly Mash	½ cup	110	1	—	—
Very Vanilla	½ cup	90	0	0	—

Sealtest Free

Chocolate, Neapolitan, Vanilla	½ cup	100	0	0	0

Sorbets

Dole

Pineapple, Raspberry	½ cup	110	<1	<1	—
Strawberry	½ cup	100	<1	<1	—

Mama Tish's

Black Raspberry, Strawberry	½ cup	100	0	0	—
Lemon	½ cup	90	0	0	0

NOTE: A dash indicates that no data are available for that food component.

(continued)

Fruit, Frozen

Food	Serving	Calories	Total Fat (g)	Saturated Fat (g)	Fiber (g)
Blackberries					
Bradys					
Whole, unsweetened	½ cup	60	<1	<1	4.0
Blueberries					
Bradys					
Unsweetened	4 oz.	60	<1	<1	3.0
Strawberries					
Whole, unsweetened (any brand)	½ cup	30	<1	<1	2.0

Mexican Foods

Food	Serving	Calories	Total Fat (g)	Saturated Fat (g)	Fiber (g)
Tortillas					
Piñata					
Corn	1 (0.9 oz.)	60	1.0	—	—

Fajita	1 (1.25 oz.)	80	2.0	—	0.5
Flour	1 (1.25 oz.)	110	2.0	—	—
Mexican Beans					
Canned Beans					
Old El Paso					
Refried Beans	½ cup	110	1.0	—	5.0
Refried Beans with Cheese	½ cup	70	2.0	2	4.0
Vegetarian Refried Beans	½ cup	140	2.0	—	10.0
Instant Beans (add water)					
Fantastic Foods					
Instant Refried Beans	½ cup	136	1.0	—	8.0
Salsas					
Chef Garcia					
Salsa, Spicy Salsa	1 oz.	6	0	0	1.0
Chi-Chi's					
Picante Salsa (mild, hot)	1 Tbsp.	6	0	0	—
Salsa (mild, medium, hot)	1 Tbsp.	4	0	0	—
Enrico					
Salsa, no salt (mild, hot)	1 Tbsp.	4	0	0	—

(continued)

Mexican Foods—Continued

Food	Serving	Calories	Total Fat (g)	Saturated Fat (g)	Fiber (g)
Salsas—Continued					
Kaukauna					
Salsa (medium, hot)	1 oz.	16	0	0	—
Miguel's					
Salsa (mild, hot)	1 Tbsp.	6	0	0	—
Newman's Own					
Bandito Mild Salsa	1 Tbsp.	6	<1	<1	—
Picante Salsa (medium, hot)	1 Tbsp.	6	<1	<1	—
Taco Salsa (mild, hot)	1 Tbsp.	6	<1	<1	—
Thick and Chunky Salsa (mild)	1 Tbsp.	4	<1	<1	—
Old Fashioned					
Hot Salsa	1 oz.	8	<1	<1	—
Chili Products					
Health Valley					
Fat-Free Mild Vegetarian Chili with 3 Beans	5 oz.	90	<1	—	9.0
Fat-Free Spicy Vegetarian Chili with Black Beans	5 oz.	140	<1	—	12.2

Mild or Spicy Vegetarian Chili with Beans	5 oz.	140	<1	—	12.2
Mild Vegetarian Chili with Lentils	5 oz.	140	3.0	—	6.8

Instant Bean Dishes*

Fantastic Foods

ChaCha Chili	10 oz.	203	2.0	—	12.0
Instant Black Beans	½ cup	136	1.0	—	8.0
Nile Spice Chili 'n Beans	7 oz.	160	1.0	—	—
Taste Adventure Red Bean Chili	6 oz.	123	1.0	—	5.0
Vegetarian Chili	½ cup	104	1.0	—	9.0

Frozen Entrées

All-Bean Products

Tumaro's

Black Bean Burrito	5 oz. (½ pkg.)	206	2.0	—	1.7
Black Bean Enchilada	5 oz. (½ pkg.)	143	2.4	—	1.7

Chicken and Beef Products

Healthy Balance

Chicken Enchilada	11 oz.	300	4.0	1	—

Healthy Choice

Beef Enchilada	12.75 oz.	350	5.0	—	—

(continued)

Mexican Foods—Continued

Food	Serving	Calories	Total Fat (g)	Saturated Fat (g)	Fiber (g)
Frozen Entrées—Continued					
Chicken and Beef Products—Continued					
Weight Watchers					
Chicken Enchiladas Suiza	9 oz.	230	7.0	2	—
Chicken Fajitas	6.75 oz.	210	5.0	2	—

*Values are for prepared dishes, with water added.

NOTE: A dash indicates that no data are available for that food component.

Muffins

Food	Serving	Calories	Total Fat (g)	Saturated Fat (g)	Fiber (g)
Ready-Made					
Health Valley					
Fat-Free Apple Spice or Raisin Spice Muffin	1	130	<1	—	5.1
Fat-Free Banana Muffin	1	130	<1	—	4.5
Fat-Free Oat Bran Fancy Fruit Muffin, Blueberry	1	140	<1	—	7.5

Food	Serving	Calories	Total Fat (g)	Saturated Fat (g)	Fiber (g)
Fat-Free Twin Pack Carrot Multi-Bran or Rasberry Muffins	1	130	<1	—	5.0
Mixes*					
Arrowhead Mills					
Oat Bran Apple Spice Muffins	1	120	4	—	5.4
Washington					
MultiBran Muffin (made with egg white)	1	120	3	<1	4.5
Oat Bran and Cinnamon Muffin (made with egg white)	1	130	4	<1	3.5

*Values are for prepared muffins.

NOTE: A dash indicates that no data are available for that food component.

Pasta and Pasta Sauces

Food	Serving	Calories	Total Fat (g)	Saturated Fat (g)	Fiber (g)
Pasta*					
Buitoni					
Spinach Linguine	8/10 cup	110	<1	<1	3.0
Deboles					
Spinach Fettuccine	8/10 cup	110	<1	<1	3.0

(continued)

Pasta and Pasta Sauces—Continued

Food	Serving	Calories	Total Fat (g)	Saturated Fat (g)	Fiber (g)
Pasta—*Continued*					
Health Valley					
100% Organic Amaranth Pasta	⁸⁄₁₀ cup	85	<1	—	4.4
100% Organic Spaghetti, Organic Spinach Spaghetti, Whole Wheat Lasagna with Wheat Germ	⁸⁄₁₀ cup	85	<1	—	3.6
Pritikin					
Whole Wheat Spaghetti	⁸⁄₁₀ cup	110	1	—	—
Westbrae					
Whole Wheat Lasagna or Spaghetti	⁸⁄₁₀ cup	110	1	—	3.5
Ramen Noodles					
Westbrae Ramen					
Buckwheat, Mushroom	1.5 oz. (½ pkg.)	150	2	—	—
Whole Wheat	1.5 oz. (½ pkg.)	170	2	—	—
Tomato Sauces					
Eden					
Spaghetti Sauce	4 oz.	80	2	—	—

Enrico					
Spaghetti Sauce, no salt added	4 oz.	60	1	—	—
Francesco Rinaldi					
Bolognese	4 oz.	60	2	0	—
Hunt's					
Mushroom	4 oz.	70	2	<1	2.0
Newman's Own					
Bandito Diavolo, Mushroom, Plain	4 oz.	70	2	—	—
Pritikin	4 oz.	60	0	0	—
Ragu					
Italian Cooking Sauce	4 oz.	70	2	—	3.0
Sauce Arturo	4 oz.	120	<1	<1	—
Weight Watchers					
Mushroom	4 oz.	40	0	0	—
Frozen Entrées					
Michelina's					
Spaghetti Marinara	10 oz.	255	2	—	—

(continued)

Pasta and Pasta Sauces—Continued

Food	Serving	Calories	Total Fat (g)	Saturated Fat (g)	Fiber (g)
Frozen Entrées—Continued					
Weight Watchers					
Angel Hair Pasta with Italian Sauce, Zucchini and Mushrooms	10 oz.	200	4	—	—

*Values are for cooked pasta.

NOTE: A dash indicates that no data are available for that food component.

Pizza, Frozen

Food	Serving (oz.)	Calories	Total Fat (g)	Saturated Fat (g)	Fiber (g)
Ellio's Healthy Slices					
Cheese	2.7	160	2	1	—
Mixed Vegetable	3.1	150	2	1	—
Healthy Choice					
Cheese	5.6	290	4	—	—

NOTE: A dash indicates that no data are available for that food component.

Rice, Barley and Other Grains

Food	Serving	Calories	Total Fat (g)	Saturated Fat (g)	Fiber (g)
Barley					
Quaker					
Scotch Brand Medium Pearled Barley	¼ cup dry	170	<1	<1	5.0
Bulgur Wheat					
Old World	¼ cup dry	150	<1	<1	3.5
Rice					
Amore Rice					
Italian Rice Arborio	1 oz. dry	90	<1	<1	1.5
Chesapeake Organic Foods					
Long Grain Brown Rice, Wild Rice Blend	½ cup	120	<1	<1	0.5
Organic Basmati Rice	½ cup	110	<1	<1	1.0
Minute					
Brown Rice	½ cup	120	1	<1	1.5
Regular Rice	½ cup	110	<1	<1	1.0

(continued)

Rice, Barley and Other Grains—Continued

Food	Serving	Calories	Total Fat (g)	Saturated Fat (g)	Fiber (g)
Rice—Continued					
Success					
Brown and Wild Rice	½ cup	120	0	0	—
Brown Rice Boil-in-Bag	½ cup	120	<1	<1	—
Texmati					
Long Grain Rice	½ cup	100	0	0	0
Uncle Ben's					
Aromatica Rice	½ cup	100	<1	<1	—
Original Fast Cooking Long Grain and Wild Rice, Original Recipe Long Grain and Wild Rice	½ cup	100	<1	<1	0.5
Long Grain Microwave Rice	½ cup	90	<1	<1	0.5
Natural Whole Grain Rice	½ cup	130	<1	<1	1.0
Rice in an Instant	½ cup	90	0	0	0.5
Rice Combinations					
Green Giant					
Rice Medley (frozen)	½ cup (4 oz.)	100	1	<1	—

Food	Serving	Calories	Total Fat (g)	Saturated Fat (g)	Fiber (g)
Success					
Beef Oriental	½ cup	100	0	0	—
Broccoli and Cheese	½ cup	120	0	0	—
Uncle Ben's					
Country Inn with Chicken Stock, Vegetable Pilaf	½ cup	120	<1	<1	0
Near East					
Lentil/Rice Pilaf	½ cup (1.1 oz. dry)	130	0	—	2.8

NOTE: A dash indicates that no data are available for that food component.

Salad Dressings

Food	Serving	Calories	Total Fat (g)	Saturated Fat (g)	Fiber (g)
Reduced-Calorie Dressings					
Hidden Valley Ranch Low-Fat					
Honey Dijon	1 Tbsp.	20	1	0	—
Italian Parmesan	1 Tbsp.	16	0	—	0
Original Ranch	1 Tbsp.	20	0	1	—

(continued)

Salad Dressings—Continued

Food	Serving	Calories	Total Fat (g)	Saturated Fat (g)	Fiber (g)
Reduced-Calorie Dressings—Continued					
Kraft					
Catalina	1 Tbsp.	18	1	0	0
French	1 Tbsp.	20	0	0	0
Kraft Free					
French, Thousand Island	1 Tbsp.	16	0	0	—
Italian	1 Tbsp.	4	0	0	—
Ranch	1 Tbsp.	18	0	0	0
Marzetti					
Light Slaw	1 Tbsp.	50	3	<1	—
Naturally Fresh					
Lite Ranch	1 Tbsp.	30	3	<1	—
Newman's Own Lite					
Reduced-Calorie Italian	1 Tbsp.	40	4	<1	0
Pfeiffer					
Caesar	1 Tbsp.	10	<1	<1	—

	Serving				
Pritikin					
French	1 Tbsp.	10	0	0	0
Italian	1 Tbsp.	6	0	0	—
Walden Farms					
Blue Cheese, Thousand Island	1 Tbsp.	25	2	—	0
French	1 Tbsp.	35	2	—	0
Italian; Italian, sodium free	1 Tbsp.	10	0	0	0
Italian, no sugar added	1 Tbsp.	6	0	0	0
Weight Watchers					
Caesar	1 Tbsp.	4	0	0	0
	1 pouch (0.75 oz.)	6	0	0	0
Creamy Ranch	1 Tbsp.	25	<1	<1	0
	1 pouch (0.75 oz.)	35	<1	<1	0
Italian	1 pouch (0.75 oz.)	6	<1	<1	0
Tomato Vinaigrette	1 Tbsp.	8	0	0	0
Regular Dressings					
Hain Italian, no salt added	1 Tbsp.	60	6	—	0
Hidden Valley Ranch					
Original Buttermilk Recipe (made from mix)	1 Tbsp.	60	3	—	0

(continued)

Salad Dressings—Continued

Food	Serving	Calories	Total Fat (g)	Saturated Fat (g)	Fiber (g)
Regular Dressings—Continued					
Kraft					
Catalina	1 Tbsp.	60	5	1	0
French, House Italian, Roka Blue Cheese	1 Tbsp.	60	6	1	0
Miracle French	1 Tbsp.	70	6	1	0
Zesty Italian	1 Tbsp.	50	5	1	0
7-Seas					
Viva Italian	1 Tbsp.	50	5	1	—
Wish-Bone					
French	1 Tbsp.	60	5	<1	0
Olive Oil Italian	1 Tbsp.	35	3	<1	—
Olive Oil Vinaigrette	1 Tbsp.	30	2	<1	—
Robusto Italian	1 Tbsp.	45	5	<1	—
Russian	1 Tbsp.	45	3	<1	—
Thousand Island	1 Tbsp.	60	6	<1	—

NOTE: A dash indicates that no data are available for that food component.

Seafood Entrées, Frozen

Food	Serving	Calories	Total Fat (g)	Saturated Fat (g)	Fiber (g)
Eating Right					
Shrimp and Vegetable Stir-Fry	9 oz.	150	4	1	—
Healthy Choice					
Linguini with Shrimp	9 oz.	270	2	1	—
Pasta with Shrimp Pasta Classic	7.9 oz.	200	4	—	—
Shrimp Creole	11.25 oz.	230	2	—	—
Shrimp Marinara	10.5 oz.	260	1	—	—
Breaded Fish Fillets	1 fillet	140	4	<1	—
Lean Cuisine					
Filet of Fish Florentine	9.6 oz.	220	7	3	—
Michelina's					
Linguini Frutti di Mare (pasta with seafood in tomato sauce)	9 oz.	260	4	—	—
Mrs. Paul's					
Light Fish Dijon	8.8 oz.	200	5	2	—

(continued)

Seafood Entrées Frozen—Continued

Food	Serving	Calories	Total Fat (g)	Saturated Fat (g)	Fiber (g)
Van de Kamp's					
Crisp and Healthy Breaded Fish Fillets	2	150	3	<1	—

NOTE: A dash indicates that no data are available for that food component.

Soups, Canned

Food	Serving (oz.)	Calories	Total Fat (g)	Saturated Fat (g)	Fiber (g)
Health Valley					
Chunky 5 Bean Vegetable Soup, no salt added	7.5	110	2	—	10.6
Chunky Vegetable Chicken Soup, no salt added	7.5	125	2	—	4.0
Fat-Free Black Bean and Vegetable Soup	7.5	70	<1	—	17.0
Fat-Free Lentil and Carrot Soup	7.5	70	<1	—	15.0
Fat-Free Real Italian Minestrone Soup	7.5	80	<1	—	4.0
Fat-Free Split Pea and Carrot Soup	7.5	50	<1	—	3.0
Fat-Free Vegetable-Barley Soup	7.5	60	<1	—	4.0
100% Natural Black Bean Soup, no salt added	7.5	150	3	—	16.9

100% Natural Lentil Soup, no salt added	7.5	170	2	—	17.0
100% Natural Minestrone Soup, no salt added	7.5	130	3	—	12.5
100% Natural Mushroom Barley Soup, no salt added	7.5	100	2	—	8.5
100% Natural Potato-Leek Soup, no salt added	7.5	130	2	—	7.4
100% Natural Split Pea Soup, no salt added	7.5	90	1	—	12.5
100% Natural Vegetable Soup, no salt added	7.5	110	1	—	8.4
Pritikin					
Lentil Soup	8.0	100	0	0	5.0
Minestrone Soup	8.0	80	<1	<1	—
Mushroom Soup	8.0	60	<1	<1	—
Navy Bean Soup	8.0	130	<1	<1	—
Split Pea Soup	8.0	140	0	0	5.0
Progresso					
Bean and Ham Soup	8.0	140	2	—	8.0
Lentil Soup	9.5	140	4	—	6.5
Manhattan Style Clam Chowder	8.0	100	2	—	8.0
Minestrone Soup	9.5	130	4	—	6.0
Vegetable Soup	8.0	60	2	—	3.5

NOTE: A dash indicates that no data are available for that food component.

(continued)

Vegetable Burger Mixes

Food	Serving (oz.)	Calories	Total Fat (g)	Saturated Fat (g)	Fiber (g)
Fantastic Foods					
Fantastic Falafel	3	129	2	—	5
Nature's Burger Barbecue	3	117	<1	—	4
Nature's Burger Original	3	152	4	—	4
Nature's Burger Pizza	3	121	1	—	4

NOTE: A dash indicates that no data are available for that food component.

Vegetables, Frozen

Food	Serving	Calories	Total Fat (g)	Saturated Fat (g)	Fiber (g)
Birds Eye					
Broccoli, Cauliflower and Red Peppers	½ cup (4 oz.)	30	0	0	3.0
Green Giant American Mixtures					
Heartland Style Broccoli, Cauliflower and Carrots	½ cup (4 oz.)	25	0	0	2.5

Food	Serving (oz.)	Calories	Total Fat (g)	Saturated Fat (g)	Fiber (g)
Broccoli Cauliflower Supreme	½ cup (4 oz.)	40	0	0	2
Green Giant Single Serve, Frozen					
Broccoli, Cauliflower and Carrots	1 pkg. (4 oz.)	25	0	0	3
Stokely Singles					
Broccoli Cauliflower	1 pkg. (3 oz.)	20	1	—	—
Broccoli, Cauliflower and Carrots	1 pkg. (3 oz.)	25	1	—	—

NOTE: A dash indicates that no data are available for that food component.

Yogurt

Food	Serving (oz.)	Calories	Total Fat (g)	Saturated Fat (g)	Fiber (g)
Colombo Lite					
All fruit flavors	8.0	190	<1	<1	—
Plain	8.0	110	<1	<1	0
Vanilla	8.0	160	<1	<1	0
Dannon					
Plain	8.0	110	0	0	0

(continued)

Yogurt—Continued

Food	Serving (oz.)	Calories	Total Fat (g)	Saturated Fat (g)	Fiber (g)
Dannon Blended					
Raspberry, Strawberry	6.0	140	0	0	—
Dannon Light*					
All fruit flavors, Cherry Vanilla, Vanilla	8.0	100	0	0	—
Mini Strawberry/Blueberry, Mini Strawberry/Peach	4.4	60	0	0	—
La Yogurt*					
Black Cherry, Strawberry, Strawberry Banana	6.0	70	0	0	0
Blueberry, Raspberry	6.0	70	0	0	0.5
Light n'Lively					
Fat-Free Strawberry Banana	4.4	50	0	0	—
Fat-Free Strawberry Fruit Cup	4.4	—	0	0	—
Stoneyfield Farm					
Nonfat Yogurt, Plain	8.0	110	0	0	0
Nonfat Yogurt, Vanilla	8.0	150	0	0	0
Nonfat Yogurt, Fruit-flavored	8.0	160	0	0	0

Weight Watchers Ultima 90					
Strawberry, Strawberry Banana	8.0	90	0	0	—
Vanilla	8.0	90	0	0	0
Yoplait*					
All fruit flavors	6.0	80	0	0	—

*These products contain NutraSweet brand sweetener.

NOTE: A dash indicates that no data are available for that food component.

Fiber Content of Popular Foods

After reading this book, you are already a fiber expert. But just for a quick refesher on foods that are high, moderate and low in fiber, you can check the tables here. The following list of great and moderate sources of fiber is not complete—there are plenty of other foods that supply healthy amounts of fiber. These are some of the most common ones.

Fiber-Rich Foods

Food	Serving	Fiber (g)
Great Sources (4 g or more)		
Brans (dry measure)		
Corn bran	⅓ cup (1 oz.)	24.0
Wheat bran	½ cup (1 oz.)	13.0
Psyllium	1 Tbsp. (⅓ oz.)	9.2

Food	Serving	Fiber (g)
Rice bran	⅓ cup (1 oz.)	6.0
Oat bran	⅓ cup (1 oz.)	4.5
Cereals and Pasta		
All-Bran with Extra Fiber	½ cup (1 oz.)	14.0
Fiber One	½ cup (1 oz.)	13.0
Bran Buds	⅓ cup (1 oz.)	11.0
All-Bran Fruit and Almond	⅔ cup (1 oz.)	10.0
100% Bran	⅓ cup (1 oz.)	10.0
All-Bran	⅓ cup (1 oz.)	9.0
Bran Flakes	⅔ cup (1 oz.)	5.0
Corn Bran	⅔ cup (1 oz.)	5.0
Bran Chex	⅔ cup (1 oz.)	4.6
Raisin Bran	¾ cup (1 oz.)	4.0–5.0
Whole wheat spaghetti, cooked	1 cup	5.9
Legumes (cooked)		
Kidney beans	½ cup	7.3
Lima beans	½ cup	6.4
Navy beans	½ cup	6.0

Moderately Rich Sources (1 to 3.9 g)
Breads and Grain Products

Whole wheat bread	1 slice	1.4
Regular spaghetti, cooked	1 cup	1.1
Brown rice, cooked	½ cup	1.0
Air-popped popcorn	1 cup	1.0

Cereals

Most	⅔ cup (1 oz.)	3.5
Toasted wheat germ	¼ cup (1 oz.)	3.4
Shredded wheat	1 biscuit (about 1 oz.)	3.0–5.0
Total (wheat)	1 cup (1 oz.)	3.0
Wheaties	1 cup (1 oz.)	3.0
Oatmeal, cooked	¾ cup	2.5
Wheat Chex	⅔ cup (1⅓ oz.)	2.1
Grape-Nuts	¼ cup (1 oz.)	1.4
Cheerios	1¼ cups (1 oz.)	1.1

(continued)

Fiber-Rich Foods—Continued

Food	Serving	Fiber (g)
Moderately Rich Sources (1 to 3.9 g)—Continued		
Fruits		
Apple	1 med.	3.5
Pear	½ large	3.1
Raisins	¼ cup	3.1
Prunes	3	3.0
Strawberries	1 cup	3.0
Orange	1 med.	2.6
Banana	1 med.	2.4
Blueberries	½ cup	2.0
Dried dates	3	1.9
Peach	1 med.	1.9
Apricots	3 med.	1.4
Cherries	10	1.2
Pineapple	½ cup	1.1
Cantaloupe	¼	1.0
Legumes and Vegetables (cooked unless otherwise specified)		
Lentils	½ cup	3.7
Green peas	½ cup	3.6
Corn	½ cup	2.9
Potato	1 med.	2.5
Brussels sprouts	½ cup	2.3
Carrot, raw	1 med.	2.3
Broccoli florets	½ cup	2.2
Spinach	½ cup	2.1
Sweet potato	½ med.	1.7
String beans	½ cup	1.6
Bean sprouts, raw	½ cup	1.5
Tomato, raw	1 med.	1.5
Kale	½ cup	1.4
Red and white cabbage, chopped	½ cup	1.4
Summer squash	½ cup	1.4
Spinach, raw	1 cup	1.2
Cauliflower florets	½ cup	1.1
Celery, raw, chopped	½ cup	1.1
Asparagus, cut	½ cup	1.0

Some foods, such as meats, dairy products, water, soft drinks and fats, contain no fiber. In addition, there are plant-based foods, such as the ones listed below, that are very low in fiber. Other than the cakes and cookies, none of these foods are high in fat, so they aren't necessarily "bad" choices. But try to make a higher-fiber choice when possible.

Fiber-Poor Foods

Food	Serving	Fiber (g)
Breads, Cereals and Grain Products		
White bread	1 slice	0.4
Corn flakes	1½ cups	0.3
Most cakes	1 slice	0.3
Most cookies	1	0.3
White rice, cooked	½ cup	0.2
Rice Krispies	1 cup	0.1
Fruits and Vegetables		
Lettuce, shredded	1 cup	0.9
Mushrooms, sliced	½ cup	0.9
Onions, sliced	½ cup	0.8
Grapes	20	0.6
Green peppers, sliced	½ cup	0.5
Watermelon chunks	1 cup	0.4
Fruit Juices		
Papaya	½ cup	0.8
Grape	½ cup	0.6
Grapefruit	½ cup	0.5
Orange	½ cup	0.5
Apple	½ cup	0.4

D

Food Diary

*K*eeping track of what you eat, when and why is a simple, practical way to analyze your eating habits, spot troublesome overeating triggers and track improvement on the Bran Plan Diet. In fact, as mentioned in chapter 8, keeping a food diary can serve as a powerful ally in your control over your eating habits.

Use the blank diary pages that follow to write down whatever you eat during the course of a few days. (Photocopy a blank page if you want to continue your diary longer.) Include important events, and plan every meal and snack as closely as possible.

Diary Page

Day:

Daily Food/ Schedule Plan (list time and event)	**What I Really Ate and Did** (list time and event and any emotions or degree of hunger)

Diary Page

Day:

**Daily Food/
Schedule Plan**
(list time and event)

What I Really Ate and Did
(list time and event and any
emotions or degree of hunger)

Diary Page

Day:

Daily Food/ Schedule Plan (list time and event)	What I Really Ate and Did (list time and event and any emotions or degree of hunger)

Diary Page

Day:

Daily Food/ Schedule Plan (list time and event)	What I Really Ate and Did (list time and event and any emotions or degree of hunger)

Diary Page

Day:

Daily Food/ Schedule Plan (list time and event)	What I Really Ate and Did (list time and event and any emotions or degree of hunger)

Diary Page

Day:

Daily Food/ Schedule Plan (list time and event)	What I Really Ate and Did (list time and event and any emotions or degree of hunger)

Diary Page

Day:

Daily Food/ Schedule Plan (list time and event)	What I Really Ate and Did (list time and event and any emotions or degree of hunger)

About the Authors

Oliver Alabaster, M.D., is a cancer researcher and practicing oncologist. He was educated at Oxford and the University of London, graduating in 1966. From 1974 until 1980 he conducted research at the National Cancer Institute, after which he served as associate professor of medicine and director of cancer research at George Washington University Medical Center in Washington, D.C.

In 1987, Dr. Alabaster established the Institute for Disease Prevention at George Washington University, where he continues to explore innovative ways to help people protect themselves against disease through dietary and lifestyle changes.

Dr. Alabaster's previous books include What You Can Do to Prevent Cancer (Simon & Schuster, 1985), later released in paperback as The Power of Prevention (Fireside Books, 1986 and Saville Books, 1988).

Janis Jibrin, R.D., is a registered dietitian and food and nutrition writer living in Washington, D.C. She is a frequent contributor to Family Circle, Self, Allure, Redbook and Longevity magazines. Ms. Jibrin has directed a number of weight-loss programs, and she counselled children with eating disorders at Georgetown University Hospital. She tests recipes for magazines and cooks for pleasure as well. Her cooking is influenced by the cuisines of various countries in which she's lived, including Greece, Italy and Lebanon.

Index

NOTE: Page references in **boldface** indicate tables.

Elderly, obesity and, 46
Emotional eating, 132–37
English muffins, brand names of,
    211–12
Estrogen
    body fat and, 44
    breast cancer and, 153
Exercise
    benefits, 54
    obesity and, 43
    overeating and, 142–43
    tips for activity, 141, 142–43
    for weight control, 48–49

F
Family, eating patterns of, 137–41
Fat, abdominal, 44
Fat, 18–28
    in American diet, 5–6, 18, 23,
        39, 47
    atherosclerosis and, 24–25
    blood pressure and, 25–26
    in breads, grains and cereals,
        reduction of, 172
    calories from, 19, 21, 45–46,
        52
    cancer and, 26–28
        colon, 13, 14
    craving for, 47
    in dairy choices, reduction of,
        162–64
    in desserts, reduction of, 170
    dietary and body, 21–22
    disease and, 18–19, 22–26
    foods containing, careful
        selection of, 166, 168
    foods high in, 40
    foods low in, 205
        brand names of, 206–55
    heart disease and, 22–26, 28
    monounsaturated, 20, 25,
        26
    overweight and, 40–41
    polyunsaturated, 20, 25, 26
    in protein sources, 165–66
    saturated, 9, 20, 22

substitutes for high-fat snacks,
    dressings, sauces and
    spreads, 169
unsaturated, 168
women's weight and, 21–22
Fatty acids, types of, 20
Fiber
    in American diet, 5–6, 16–17
    benefits, 5–17
    for cancer prevention, 12–15
    for diabetes, 16
    dietary requirements, 16–17,
        32
        Fiber Intake Quiz, 32–35
    disease and, 6–8, 12–16
    for diverticular disease and
        irritable colon, 15
    foods high in, 205
        brand names of, 206–55
    for gallstones, 16
    for heart attack and stroke
        prevention, 9–12
    for hemorrhoids and varicose
        veins, 15
    for obesity, 16
    in popular foods, 256–59
    types, 8
Fish. See also Seafood
    Broiled Fish with Garlic-
        Lemon Marinade, 197
    low-fat, as protein source, 165
    omega-3 fatty acids in, 20–21
    Salmon Salad, 192–93
    Tropical Glazed Fish, 197
    Tuna Salad, 194
Flatulence, from fiber, 8
Folic acid, in diet, 149
Food portions
    controlling, 129
    in Lifelong Bran Plan, 157–62
    measurement conversions for,
        63
Foods
    avoiding, 140
    in Bran Plan Diet, 3–4
    craving, 132–37

Lentils
portions in Lifelong Bran
Plan, 161
Thick Lentil Soup, 175
Lifelong Bran Plan, 154–72
adding phase, 156–57
calorie levels in, 155, **156**
steps in, 154
substitution phase, 162
Lifestyle, obesity and, 41–42
Lipoproteins, HDL vs. LDL, 23
Lung cancer, cruciferous vegetables
and, 153

M
Marinades
Broiled Fish with Garlic-
Lemon Marinade, 197
Tropical Glazed Fish, 197
Measurement conversions for food
portions, 63
Meat, lean
cooking, 167
as protein source, 164–65
Men, overweight and, 43–44, 45
Menopause, fat accumulation after,
44–45
Menu plans for weight loss, 59–63
Cook's Plan, 59, 60, **64–92**
Take-Out Plan, 59, 60,
93–122
Metabolism
Bran Plan for Weight Loss
and, 51
obesity and, 42–43, 49
yo-yo dieting and, 51, 55
Metamucil, 31
Mexican foods, 186
All-Bean Chili, 188
Bean Burrito, 187
brand names of, **234–38**
Chicken Fajita, 186
Fresh Tomato Salsa, 189
A Mano's Tropical Salsa, 189
Refried Beans, 187

Milk, in weight-loss menus, 61
Minerals, toxicity of, 148
Mineral supplements, 146–48
for Bran Plan for Weight Loss,
59–60
Mint
Mint-Yogurt Topping, 203
Motivational strategies for
overeating, 124–43
Muffins
brand names of, **238–39**
Homemade Muffins, 182

N
Niacin, in diet, 149
Night blindness, from vitamin A
deficiency, 147
Nutrition, in Bran Plan, 4, 144–53
Nuts and seeds, in Lifelong Bran
Plan, 168

O
Oat bran
in Bran Cocktail, 30, 31
cholesterol lowered by, 10, 12
Obesity, 40. *See also* Bran Plan for
Weight Loss; Overweight;
Weight control and loss
aging and, 46
fiber for, 16
genetic factors, 41–43
Omega-3 fatty acids, 20–21
cancer protection from, 27–28
Oranges and orange juice, for
longevity, 152–53
Overeating, controlling, 123–43
dealing with family, 137–41
exercise, 142–43
food cravings or emotional
eating, 132–37
food/schedule diary, 125,
126, 127, 260–67
identifying obstacles, 128
social eating, 128–32
weight scale, 127

Rice
    Bran Cocktail Brown Rice,
        181
    brand names of, **243–45**
    Lentil-Barley Pilaf, 180
    Shellfish Risotto, 200–201
    Tomato Rice, 181
Rickets, from vitamin D deficiency,
    150
Rolls, brand names of, **212**

S
Salad dressings, 190
    Basic Vinaigrette, 191
    brand names of, **245–48**
    high-fat, substitutes for, **169**
    Honey-Mustard Vinaigrette,
        191
    Raspberry Topping for Fruit
        Salad, 190
    Tangerine Vinaigrette, 192
Salads, 192
    Carrot-Cabbage Coleslaw,
        193
    Mixed Greens Salad, 195
    Salmon Salad, 192–93
    Spinach Salad, 194
    Three-Bean Salad, 177
    Tomato-Cucumber Salad, 195
    Tuna Salad, 194
Salmon
    Pasta with Smoked Salmon
        and Watercress, 199
    Salmon Salad, 192–93
Salsas
    A Mano's Tropical Salsa, 189
    Black Bean and Dried Fruit
        Salsa, 176–77
    Fresh Tomato Salsa, 189
Sauces
    Basil-Tomato Sauce, 185
    high-fat, substitutes for, **169**
    tomato, brand names of,
        240–41

Scale, weight control and, 127
Scallops
    Shellfish Risotto, 200–201
Scurvy, from vitamin C deficiency,
    146–47, 149
Seafood
    brand names of, **249–50**
    Broiled Fish with Garlic-
        Lemon Marinade, 197
    Craig Claiborne's Linguine
        with Clam Sauce, 198
    dishes, 196
    Grilled Shrimp with Hot and
        Sweet Red Peppers, 196
    Pasta with Smoked Salmon
        and Watercress, 199
    Salmon Salad, 192–93
    Shellfish Risotto, 200–201
    Tropical Glazed Fish, 197
    Tuna Salad, 194
Seeds and nuts, in Lifelong Bran
    Plan, 168
Selenium, in diet, 151
Shrimp
    Grilled Shrimp with Hot and
        Sweet Red Peppers, 196
Skim milk, in weight-loss menus,
    61
Skin cancer, garlic and, 152
Snacks
    in Lifelong Bran Plan, 160,
        170–71
    high-fat, substitutes for,
        169
Social eating, 128–32
Sorbets, brand names of, **233**
Soups
    brand names of, **250–51**
    Thick Lentil Soup, 175
Soybeans, for longevity, 153
Spinach
    Spinach Salad, 194
Spreads, high-fat, substitutes for,
    169

Vitamin supplements, 146–48
    for Bran Plan for Weight Loss,
        59–60

W

Waist-to-hip ratio as indicator of
    health risks, 40, 44
Walking, for exercise, 141
Water, with fiber intake, 35
Watercress
    Pasta with Smoked Salmon
        and Watercress, 199
Water weight, 127
Weight control and loss. *See also*
    Overeating, controlling
        Bran Plan for, 3
            Cook's Plan, 59, 60,
                63–92
            menu plans, 59–63
            Take-Out Plan, 59, 60,
                93–122, 140

calories and, 54–55
dietary fat and, 21–22
Wheat bran, 12
    in Bran Cocktail, 30, 31
Women, overweight and, 43–45

Y

Yogurt
    Banana Shake, 203
    brand names of, **253–55**
    frozen, **231–32**
    Mint-Yogurt Topping, 203
    recipes, 202
    Yogurt-Dill Topping, 204
    Yogurt Topping for Fruit, 204
Yo-yo dieting, 2, 46, 47–48
    metabolism and, 51, 55

Z

Zinc absorption, 146